BASIC PRINCIPLES OF NUTRITION

BASIC PRINCIPLES OF NUTRITION

SEEMA YADAV

ANMOL PUBLICATIONS PVT. LTD.
NEW DELHI - 110 002 (INDIA)

ANMOL PUBLICATIONS PVT. LTD.
4374/4B, Ansari Road, Daryaganj
New Delhi - 110 002
www.anmolbooks.com

Basic Principes of Nutrition

First Edition, 1997
Reprint, 2002

ISBN 81-7488-534-X

PRINTED IN INDIA

Published by J.L. Kumar for Anmol Publications Pvt. Ltd., New Delhi - 110 002 and Printed at Mehra Offset Press, Delhi.

Contents

Contents

Preface

The book has been written primarily to serve as a text book. The book presents the matter with the assumption that the students entering the college these days leave a good knowledge of basic sciences and it is with this assumption in mind that the simplified approach has not been adopted. The book can be quite helpful to the professional nutritionist as various aspects of nutrition discussed in the book have to be used by such persons. The statistical data presented in the book is also of much help to such persons.

An attempt has been made in this book to consolidate the fundamentals of nutritions with recent advances in the field. The book provides a unified picture of nutrition and its principles laying special emphasis on nutrients present in food, their functions, their requirements, their metabolism, the diseases caused due to their deficiency, the sources of various nutrients and how to make further improvements in the nutrients in diet.

For preparing the book I have used the material published in various and author expresses my gratitude to all such publishers whose material has been used. I would also like to thank some of my friends for making quite useful suggestions during the preparation of manuscript.

Suggestions for any improvement in the book shall be gratefully appreciated.

Author

1

Introduction to Nutrition

1.1. General Introduction

Among various modern developments that have added to our insight into the processes of life, enabling us to understand these processes better, and increasingly to control and improve them, one of the most important is the chemistry of food and nutrition.

Nutrition is the science of nourishing the body and the nutritive substance for his purpose are provided by **Food**. Thus *Nutrition is the science that interprets the relationship of food to the functioning of living organisms.* It includes the uptake of food, liberation of energy, elimination of wastes, and all the enzymes essential for maintenance, growth and reproduction.

Nutrition is a relatively new science that evolved from chemistry and physiology, just as biophysics has more recently evolved, from biology and physics.

1.2. Historical Aspects

Beginning of the Study of Nutrition

The desire to probe the mysteries of nourishment is an old one and the search has continued ever since the times immemorial.

In the first century B.C. it was common belief in Egypt that the cause of many a diseases is excessive eating. The Greek philosopher Hippocrates (460-359 B.C.) observed and stated, "Growing bodies have the most innate heat; they require the most food otherwise their bodies are wasted. In old people the heat is feable and they require little fuel, as it were, for it would be extinguished by much."

Another important observation made by him is, "Persons who are naturally very fat are apt to die earlier than those who are slender."

Some of the statements made by Leonardo de Vinci (1452-1519) have a modern connotation. About the need for nourishment be observed.

... if you do not supply nourishment equal to the nourishment departed, life will fail in vigor; and if you take away this nourishment, life is utterly destroyed.

The need for oxygen—where flame cannot live no animal can sustain its existence.

Studies on Respiration: In the beginning of seventeenth century the mysteries of "air" and of processes of respiration were under investigation. Most significant were the experiments of John Mayow (1643-1679). He placed a small animal and a burning candle in a closed jar. He observed that the candle burned a longer time without the animal in the jar, and that the animal lived a longer time in the jar without the burning candle. Mayowat at the age of 25 wrote a treatise on respiration. With perceiving vision he stated that "the particles of the air absorbed during respiration are designed to convert the black or venous blood into the red or arterial." This young scientist died when he was only 36, cutting short his brilliant career.

For about a century no progress was made in the field and it was after the lapse of such a long period following discoveries made in about 15-20 years laid the ground work for the science of nutrition.

About a century elapsed before others took up the studies respiration. In a period of about 15 years four men were born who made discoveries that laid the groundwork for the science of nutrition.

Joseph Black (1728-1799), a physician and professor at the university of Edinburgh, discovered what he termed "fixed air," later identified as carbon dioxide. He found that by breathing through a tube into lime water, it became cloudy; also when poured into a jar in which a candle had been burned, the lime water became cloudy. Black proposed that all kinds of animals expire "fixed air."

Joseph Priestly (1733-1804) and Karl Scheele (1742-1786) independently discovered oxygen at about the same time. Priestley was a Unitarian clergyman in England, Scheele a Swedish apothecary and chemist.

Priestley thought that both animals and flames exhausted the air. He wondered how the air once "exhausted" could be revitalized. He found the answer by burning a candle in a jar until it went out, and then placing a living plant (a sprig of mint) in the jar. Ten, days later he placed another candle in the enclosed space and found that it burned perfectly well; the living plant had revitalized the air. Priestley produced oxygen by heating red oxide of mercury in a closed vessel with the heat of the sun focused by means of burning glass.

Scheele performed an experiment in which he placed two large bees with a little honey in a small box fitted in the top of a glass cylinder. He immersed the cylinder in limewater after filling it with "fire-air" (his term for oxygen), that he had obtained by heating mercuric oxide. After eight days the bees were both dead and the limewater had risen in the container. The "fire-air" had been used up by the bees and the carbon dioxide give off was absorbed in the limewater.

It was Lavoisier who explained the phenomenon of respiration. In 1762, he stated. " Respiration is only a slow combustion of carbon and hydrogen which is entirely similar to that which obtains in a lamp or lighted candle and from this point of view aniwals which respire are truely combustible bodies which burn and consume themselves. In respiration as in combustion, it is the air which furnishes the oxygen— but in respiration it is the body substance which furnishes the heat— if animals do not repair constantly the losses of respiration, the lamp soon lacks oil, and animal dies, as a lamp goes out when it lacks food."

Lavoisier however did not recognize the nature of food stuffs and believed that elemental carbon and hydrogen were oxidized in the body. Magendie (1783-1855) was first to distinguish between the different kinds of food stuffs, (carbohydrates, Fats, proteins). Form his experiment on dog he concluded that the protein element was necessary. However even this information was not applied to the study of respiratory exchange for many years. Regnault and Rieset is 1840 showed that the ratio of carbon dioxide expired to oxygen consumed varied with the kind of food. This ratio is now called the *Respiratory Quotient* (R.Q.)

Calorimetric Studies

In the twentieth century a lot of knowledge has been gained about nutrition. The calorimetric studies carried out at the beginning of this century clearly established a relationship between energy and nutrition. Later experiments were able to correlate the nutritional functions of proteins and it was found that food proteins or their amino acids are the antecedents and precursors of many of the body's catalysts which are necessary for the chemical reactions involved in digestion and nutrition. During last 30-40 years there has come an awakening to the importance mineral elements is nutrition and the nutritive value of foods. If has now been established that these elements are essential.

The vitamins as a class are the other compounds whose importance in nutrition is now well established. Between 1930 and 1940 the majority of vitamins were identified, isolated from foods and synthesized is the laboratory. With this knowledge it became possible to develop a completely synthetic diet. This work provided the basic information that is the core of the science of nutrition.

The twentieth century ushered in the "one world" concept also and with it, concern not only for an adequate diet for our nation, but for enough food to feed the world. Some of the scientists and certain of their contributions will be referred to in the chapters to follow.

Some Important Definitions

Food : It is a kind of fuel for living things.

Fortified Food : It has had added to it nutrients such as vitamins or other dietary essentials in amount sufficient to make the total content greater than the natural (unprocessed) food of its class, as in the addition of vitamin D to milk.

Metabolism : The change which takes place in the food stuffs, after they have been absorbed from the digestive tract.

Nutrition : It is the functional aspect of food chemistry.

Functions of Food

(*i*) It provides energy to do work and to maintain body heat.

(*ii*) It provides material for the growth of the body.

(*iii*) It provides material for the repair of damaged cells and tissues of our body.

(*iv*) It makes materials necessary for reproduction.

(*v*) It regulates body processes to maintain life.

Even though the chief functions of food are the ones listed above (physiological functions) but food also plays an integral role in social life. It also has the psychological or emotional influence which may be considered as its function.

Social Functions of Food

To serve food at many social functions in quite prevalent in our country. Such functions are marriage, birth day etc. Even high dignitaries arrange social get togethers on certain religious occasion such as Id etc. All these social gatherings where we serve sumptuous food to our guests indirectly serve as an instrument to develop social rapport. The main criterion of selection of food items to be served at such social gatherings in schools, colleges or even at other functions is not the nutritive value of the food item but its popularity with the guests.

Psychological Functions of Food

Food satisfies certain emotional needs in our social life. Even though a meal may be adequate nutritionally, it may not give a sense of genuine satisfaction. People who travel or live in a new land often find adjusting to the unfamiliar food customs a problem. With time the strange becomes familiar and new likes are formed. Traditional habits are characterized by certain foods pleasing persons of one culture and being distasteful to those of another.

Food is also used to express feelings. The giving of food is token of friendship; the serving of favorite foods an expression of special attention and recognition; and the withholding of wanted foods a means of punishment.

2

The Carbohydrates

2.1. Introduction

Carbohydrates serve a unique function in nature as they are the chief source of nutriment for the animal kingdom. This nutrient is the main source of energy for the people of the world. The rice, cassava, sugars, potatoes, corn, wheat and other cereal grains are rich sources of carbohydrates.

All carbohydrates contain carbon, hydrogen and oxygen. In a simple carbohydrate unit, there are six carbon atoms arranged in a chain with atoms of hydrogen and oxygen attached to the carbons in the same ratio as found in water, two to one. The chemical formula of glucose is presented in Fig. 2.1. The energy value of carbohydrates is 4 Cal. of energy per gram of the nutrient.

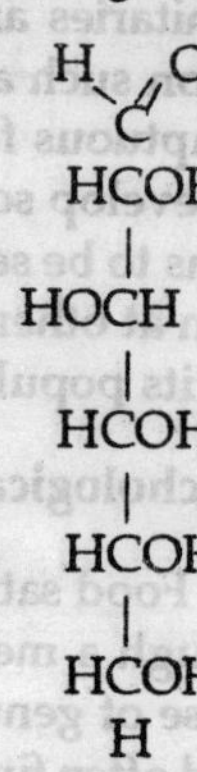

fIg. 2.1. The chemical formula of glucose.

Of the various constituents of the ordinary food of man, the carbohydrates are generally the most abundant and the most economical sources of energy. They are also considered to be the first of the three great groups of organic foodstuffs to be formed by synthesis from simple inorganic substances in plants: "in the long run, all the energy of living matter comes from them." The synthesis of carbohydrates in nature is therefore a logical starting point for the study of the organic foodstuffs.

Green leaves utilize the radiant energy of sunshine to bring about the process of *photosynthesis* wherein organic compounds like sugars and starches are synthesized from carbon dioxide and water. Thus is "bound" or "stored" energy that later becomes available when any direct or indirect product of photosynthesis is used up as a fuel foodstuff in the body.

We here review only the few carbohydrates most important in food and nutrition and those only in their simplest relations.

2.2. Classification of Carbohydrates

Carbohydrates are defined an polyhydroxy aldehydes and ketones and vary from simple there carbon sugars to relatively complex polymers. Older definitions that precisely relate the ratio of carbon, hydrogen and oxygen in the molecule are no longer valid. The general classification of carbohydrates includes compounds that are not true hydrates e.g. deoxyribose and a large number of derivatives of saccharides as well.

A simple classification of some carbohydrates important in nutrition, based on the number of single carbohydrates units found in each chemical structure, is shown in Fig. 2.2. Compounds having one carbohydrates units are known as *monosaccharides*, those with two units are called *disaccharides,* and compounds with more than two carbohydrates units are called polysaccharides

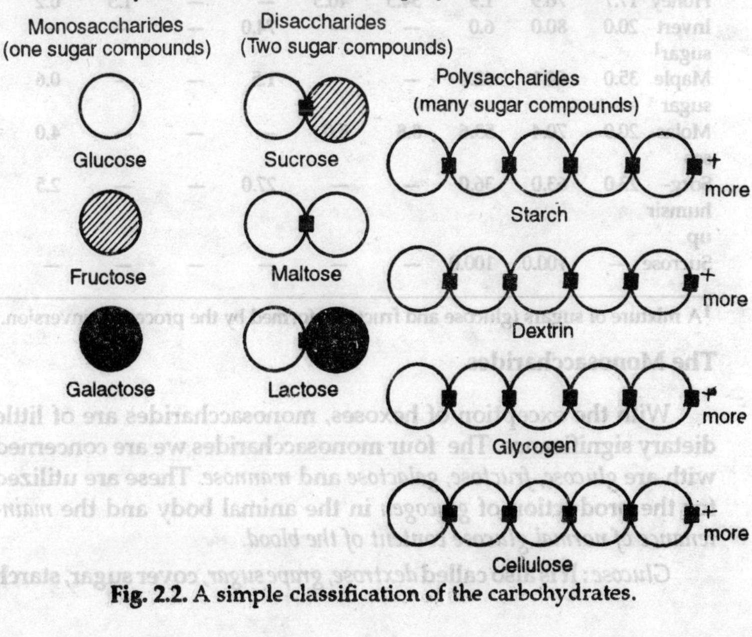

Fig. 2.2. **A simple classification of the carbohydrates.**

Most of the mono- and disaccharides are soluble in water, crystalline in structure, and have a sweet taste; they are known as sugars and are having a characteristic name ending, *-ose*. However, most polysaccharides are insoluble in water and they do not form crystals, do not have a taste sweet, and have neither a group name nor a characteristic ending. The approximate composition of various sweetening agents is presented in Table 2.1.

Table 2.1. Approximate Composition of Various Sweetening Agents, in Percentage

Sugar Product	*Water*	*Total Sugar*	*Sucrose*	*Dextrose*	*Levulose*	*Invert Sugar*[1]	*Maltose*	*Dextrins*	*Ash*
Corn sirup	17.7	47.6	—	21.2	—	—	26.4	34.7	—
Corn sugar (cerelose)	9.0	91.6	—	87.5	—	--	3.5	0.5	0.04
Gloden sirup	22.5	68.5	31.0	—	—	37.5	—	—	3.9
Honey	17.7	76.9	1.9	34.5	40.5	—	—	1.5	0.2
Invert sugar[1]	20.0	80.0	6.0	—	—	74.0	—	—	—
Maple sugar	35.0	64.1	62.6	—	—	1.5	—	—	0.6
Molasses	20.0	70.4	53.6	8.8	8.0	—	—	—	4.0
Sorghumsirup	23.0	63.0	36.0	—	—	27.0	—	—	2.5
Sucrose	—	100.0	100.0	—	—	—	—	—	—

[1] A mixture of sugars (glucose and fructose) formed by the process of Inversion.

The Monosaccharides

With the exception of hexoses, monosaccharides are of little dietary significance. The four monosaccharides we are concerned with are *glucose*, *fructose*, *galactose* and *mannose*. These are utilized for the production of *glycogen* in the animal body and the *maintenance of normal glucose content of the blood*.

Glucose: It is also called *dextrose*, *grape sugar*, cover sugar, starch sugar, diabetic sugar and is widely distributed in nature.

Sources

Plant kingdom : Fruits, vegetables and sap. corn sugar, corn sirup, honey, molasses.

Animals : In the animal body it is an end product of digestion of starch, sucrose, maltose and lactose.

In the healthy body the glucose of the blood is constantly being burned and replaced. Ordinarily any surplus of glucose absorbed from the digestive tract is converted into glycogen which, is readily reconvertible into glucose. Thus, while other carbohydrates occur in food in greater quantity, glucose occupies a very prominent place, partly because it is so widely distributed in both plants and animals, and partly because it is the form in which most of the carbohydrate material of the food comes actually into the service of the body. It is estimated that (under ordinary conditions) over half the energy manifested in the human body is in this sense derived from the oxidation of glucose.

Man's normal level of blood glucose is about 80 mg of glucose per 100 ml of blood and is maintained within a narrow range by the balance of glucose entering and leaving the blood stream. Blood glucose originates from dietary carbohydrate, from stores of glycogen, or from carbohydrate synthesis. In diabetes, a disorder caused by the body's inability to use glucose, the blood glucose level is elevated.

Fructose : It is also called *fruit sugar, levulose.*

Sources : Plant juices, fruits, honey.

In honey it constitutes about are half of the solid matter.

It serves, like glucose, for the production of *glycogen*.

Glucose and fructose are interconvertible. In liver, fructose gets converted to glycogen and glycogen hydrolysis yields glucose.

The interconversion of glucose and fructose occurs through the intermediate formation of a dienol (ene - diol).

Galactose : It does not occur free in nature and is produced in the body during the digestion of disaccharides such as lactose. If the individual is lacking in an enzyme that converts galactose to glucose he is likely to suffer from *galactosemia* (an infant disease).

Polymeric anhydrides of galactose, known as galactans, occur quite widely distributed in plants; and galactosides, which are compounds containing galactose in chemical combination with radicles of other than carbohydrate nature, are constituents of the brain and nerve tissues. Galactose has been recognized as a minor constituent of several proteins.

Mannose also, although not prominent in the carbohydrate food-stuffs, has recently been reported as occurring (in traces) in several proteins.

Disaccharides

All the three disaccharides considered here are *dihexoses* or *hexobioses* represented by the chemical formula $C_{12} H_{22} O_{11}$. They are all crystallizable and readily diffusible. They are *sucrose, lactose* and *maltose.*

Sucrose : It is the sugar that we use in our daily life which is generally obtained from sugar cane and sugar beets. It also occurs in some fruits and vegetables. It is commonly found in sweetening agents. Maple sirup and molasses contain more than 50% sucrose. Small quantities of it are also found to occur in sorghum sirup, golden sirup and honey. It forms glucose and fructose when hydrolyzed during digestion.

The hydrolysis of sucrose is to change the sign ("invert") of rotation from + to - and for this reason it is called *inversion* and the resulting mixture containing equal quantities of glucose and fructose is known as *invert sugar.*

The hydrolysis takes place in stomach in the presence of hydrochbric acid.

Lactose : It is also called *milk sugar* and occurs in the milk of all mammals. Its amount is about 7% in human milk and 5% in cow or goat milk. It is believed that it is formed in the mammary glands from the glucose brought by the blood.

It is less sweet and only slightly soluble in water on hydrolysis by heating with acid or by an enzyme (e.g. *lactose*) it yields glucose and fructose (1 molecule each). It is less subject to fermentation in the stomach than sucrose.

Recent research carried out by Associates of Rogers (1935), has shown that the taking of liberal quantities of lactose in the food is for some people an important aid to the maintenance of good intestinal conditions because the lactose is especially favourable to the development of desirable types of intestinal bacteria, notably the *Bacillus (Lactobacillus) acidophilus.*

In order that this latter advantage may be had along with greater solubility and apparent sweetness for those who desire it, *betalactose** has been studied scientifically and made commercially available.

Maltose : It is also called *milk sugar* and is formed from starch by the action diastatic enzyme (e.g. *amylases*). It is an important constituent of germinating cereals, malt and malt products. The most important source of maltose for the body is an intermediate product of starch digestion. It is also formed as an intermediate product when starch is digested in the human or other animal body, or hydrolyzed by boiling with dilute mineral acid as in the manufacture of commercial glucose.

In animal digestion, maltose is formed by the action of the ptyalin of the saliva (salivary amylase) or of the amylopsin of the pancreatic juice (pancreatic amylase) upon starch or dextrin. The maltose-splitting enzyme of the intestinal juice readily hydrolyzes maltose to glucose. Maltose is also readily and completely hydrolyzed by boiling with dilute mineral acids on hydrolysis it yields two molecules of glucose.

Polysaccharides

The polysaccharides are complex carbohydrates that may contain as many as 2000 simple carbohydrate units arranged in long chains in either a straight or a branched structure. Starch, dextrin, glycogen, and cellulose are four polysaccharides that are important in the study of nutrition.

Starch and glycogen are the typical reserve carbohydrates of plants and animals respectively. The dextrins are the intermediate products in the hydrolysis of starch.

Starch : It is he most important carbohydrate is man's diet. It is stored in the plants (roots, seeds and tubers) as $(C_6H_{10}O_5)_n$. It

---

\# Lactose, Glucose-β-galactoside, exists in α- and β-forms corresponding to α- and β-glucose. The ordinary "milk sugar" of commerce is α-lactose. However by allowing solutions of lactose to crystallize above 90°, the β-isomer is obt-

is an important source of dextrins, maltose and glucose.

The seeds of plants are nature's richest storehouses of starch. Corn, millet, rice, rye, and wheat, the important cereal grains, contain as much as 70 per cent of this carbohydrate, whereas the percentage of starch found in the dried seeds of leguminous plants (e.g., beans, peas) averages about 40 per cent.

Starch is found in the cells of pants in the form of granules. These granules, different in size and shape and markings, are typical of the plants in which they occur. Wheat starch granules are oval-shaped; the granules of cornstarch are small, rounded and angular.

Starch granules are not affected by cold water; on warming they absorb water and swell. Finally, the starch changes into a colloidal dispersion or semi-solution, "starch paste." Starch that has been heated in water (either admixed or naturally present with the starch as in a potato) until the granules are ruptured and the material more or less dispersed is much more rapidly hydrolyzed by digestive enzymes than is raw starch. The starch-digesting enzymes *(amylases)* of the saliva and pancreatic juice change starch through dextrin to maltose; and a digestive ferment of the intestinal juice changes the maltose to glucose.

In starch cookery, as the temperature of the liquid increases, the granules begin to swell and mixture becomes viscous; this change is called *gelatinization*. Cooking makes starch-containing foods more palatable and more easily digested. Glucose is the end product of all starch hydrolyzed in the body.

Dextrins : Their formula is $(C_6 H_{10} O_5)_n$ or $(C_6 H_{10} O_5)_n H_2O$. They occurs as metabolic products in animals and plants and are much more abundant in germinating seeds. *Malt diastase* (an enzyme) hydrolyses a concentrated solution of starch to yields dextrin and dextrins formed in this way are called *hydrolytic dextrins.*

Commercial dextrin which is the principal constituent of "British gum" is obtained by heating starch and the dextrins formed by dry heating are called *torrefaction dextrins.*

They are more soluble than starch. On complete hydrolysis they produce glucose. The work of Rettger indicates that dextrin is, like lactose, a favourable medium for a nourishment of the *Lactobacillus acidophilus* in the digestive tract, so that liberal proportions of dextrin and lactose in the food are conducive to a good intestinal hygiene.

Glycogen : It is represented by the formula $(C_6 H_{10} O_5)_n$. Its role in animals is quite similar to that of starch in plants and for this reason it is called *animal starch.*

It is formed in liver of all animals and in small aquatic animals called mussels.

It is a white amorphous power that is odorless and tasteless. It swells and *terms* dissolves in cold water to form a colloidal dispersion that is not cleared by repeated filtration, but loses its opalescence on addition of a very small amount of potassium hydroxide or acetic acid. Water solutions (dispersions) of glycogen get readily precipitated by alcohol. When treated with iodine they form yellow-brown, red-brown, or deep red. Complete hydrolysis of glycogen yields glucose only.

Muscle glycogen, which represents about two-thirds of the total reserve, is designated solely for the use of muscle tissue whereas liver glycogen is available as a source of energy to any of the body cells.

The formation and breakdown or glycogen in the body, which involve a series of complex chemical reactions, are directly related to several physiological factors. (The formation of glycogen takes place when the blood glucose in increased beyond its normal level and extra amounts of glucose are present in the blood stream). In contrast the breakdown of glycogen takes place when carbohydrate is not being absorbed from the intestinal tract, and to meet this deficit the emergency supply of body energy, liver glycogen must be utilized until the cell can begin to synthesize glucose from non- carbohydrate sources (*glyconeogenesis*).

Cellulose: It is the constituent of cell walls of plants cell. Though it is of little nutritive value but its presence in proper proportion in the diet as a whole is favourable to the mechanics of digestion and the hygiene of digestive tracts. Those materials which are not dissolved by the digestive enzymes are known as "Roughages". *Roughages* are important in the diet of man to help in the maintenance of the normal peristaltic action of the intestines and in the removal of waste product from the intestinal tract. This polysaccharide is an important a source of roughage to the intestinal tract which absorbs moisture and provides bulk to stimulate the normal evacuation of the large intestine.

The best food sources of cellulose or fiber are dried fruits whole-grain cereals, nuts, fresh fruits, and vegetables. Milk, meat, eggs, cheese, and highly refined foods (e.g., white flour and sugar) are poor in fiber. Because the fiber in meat is protein, it is digestible and provides little if any bulk to the intestinal tract. We can estimate the fiber content of a diet and the daily need for fibre is, estimated to be 4 to 7 mg which may be easily obtained if the diet includes a serving of whole-grain cereal or bread, two servings of vegetables, and two servings of fruit.

Hetero polysaccharides : The mucopolysaccharides (sometimes called heteropolysaccharides) are heteropolysaccharides and occur in combination with protein in both body secretions and structures. Many mucopolysaccharides tend to be highly viscous and are responsible for the viscosity of body mucous secretions. Although the axact structure of many of these compounds is uncertain, they have been identified by the products they yields an hydrolysis.

2.3. Functions of Carbohydrates

Carbohydrates are the main source of energy in our food. The starch and sugar provide most of the energy (60 - 80 %) to our body. They are the cheapest source of energy though the fats are the richest source of energy.

In addition to providing energy carbohydrates also help in the utilization of body fats. It also exert a sparing effect as proteins and plays an important role in functions of intestinal tract. It also adds flavour to the diet.

The expression 'fat burns in a flame of carbohydrates' is generally used to sum up the role of carbohydrates in utilization of body fats. Complete oxidation of fats to the metabolic end products of carbon dioxide and water depends on an organic acid, pyruvic acid, produced during the oxidation for carbohydrates. When insufficient quantities of carbohydrates are available, greater than normal amounts of ketone bodies are formed. The accumulation of ketone bodies increases the acidity and reduces the alkalinity of the blood. This condition, known as *ketosis,* may result in a coma if the alkalinity of the blood is reduced appreciably.

Ketosis may occur in diabetes where the cells fail to utilize carbohydrate and in starvation where the cells must use the fat stores of the body for energy.

2.4. Carbohydrates in the Worlds' Food Supply

Since carbohydrates are the main source of food energy so we give here. (in tabular form) the percentage of carbohydrates in some typical foods (Table 2.2). The total calories derived from cereals, starchy roots and sugars as a percentage of total food calories for various region of the world are listed in Table 2.3.

Table 2.2. The Percentage of Carbohydrate in Some Typical Foods

Carbohydrate	*The Foods*			
Per cent				
between	brown sugar			
100-91	white sugar			
90-81	corn flakes	marshmallows		
	honey	peanut butter		
	maple sugar	rice cereals		
	bran flakes	dates	popcorn	wheat flakes
80-71	cookies	fudge	shredded wheat	
	crackers	oat cereals	sirups	
	chocolate sirup		molasses	
70-61	dried apricots			
	jellies and jams			
	cakes		white bread	
60-51	chocolate bars			
	dried nonfat milk solids			
	potato chips			
50-41	rolls			
	whole-wheat bread			
	apple pie			

(Contd.)

40-31	French fried potatoes			
	sweet potatoes			

	baked potato			
30-21	banana			
	cooked	macaroni noodles	rice	spaghetti
	apple	ice cream	peas	
20-11	corn	Lima beans		
	grapes	pears		
	beef liver	carrot	green beans	orange
10-0	broccoli	Cheddar cheese	melons	peaches
	butter	egg	milk	tomatoes
	beef	lamb veal		
none	chicken	pork		
	fats oils	salmon		

Table 2.3. Calories Derived from Cereals, Starchy Roots, and Sugar as a Percentage of Total Food Calories Available throughout the World

	Percentage derived
Africa:	
East and southern Africa	73
North Africa	75
West and central Africa	74
Asia:	
China, mainland	83
Eastern Asia	80
Near East	72
South Asia	78
Southeastern Asia, mainland	78
Southeastern Asia, major islands	81
Europe:	
Eastern Europe and U.S.S.R.	71
Western Europe	55

(Contd.)

Oceania:	
Australia and New Zealand	48

North America:	
Canada and United States	40
Caribbean	60
Central America	71
Mexico	85
South America:	
Brazil	64
North and western countries	66
River Plate countries	54

An analysis of the results tabulated in Table 2.3 shows that African countries derive 74% of their total calories from carbohydrates and in Asia it ranges from 72-83%. Similar percentages can be seen for some other regions. e.g.

Near East countries	—	72 %
Far East countries	—	81 %
West European countries	—	55 %
East European countries	—	71 %
Canada and U.S.A.	—	40 %
Mexico	—	85 %

In "high calorie countries" (i.e. Canada, Europe, Oceania, River Plate countries, U.S.A.) about 57% of energy is obtained from cereals etc. Where as in low calori countries (i.e. Africa, Far east, Latin America and Near East) about 78% of energy comes from same food (i.e. cereals, starchy roots and sugars).

If one consider the whole world average of energy obtained from such carbohydrates foods it comes out to be 70% of the total calories.

3

Fats and Lipids

3.1. Introduction

Lipids are one of the large group of organic compounds which are of great importance in food we eat. Fats are readily digested and utilized in the body. They are widely distributed in natural foods. Even fruits and vegetables which are not considered as sources of fats and lipids also contain about 0.1 - 0.2 % of it.

The lipids are characterized by their solubility in ether, chloroform, benzene and other fat solvents. They contain carbon, hydrogen and oxygen. In some lipids nitrogen and phosphorus are also present.

Bloor (1943) used the term *Lipids* to cover the fats and related substances and defined *lipids* as naturally occurring substances consisting of higher fatty acids, their naturally occurring compounds found in natural association with them.

3.2. Classification of Lipids

The lipids are classified into three groups according to their chemical structure—

1. The simple lipids
2. The compounds lipids, and
3. The derived lipids.

Bloor's Classification of Lipids

Simple lipids : Esters of the fatty acids with various alcohols. Fats—esters of the fatty acids with glycerol.

Waxes—ester of the fatty acids with alcohols* other than glycerol.

Compounds lipids : Esters of the fatty acids containing groups in addition to an alcohol and fatty acid.

Phospholipids (phosphatides)—substituted fats containing phosphoric acid and nitrogen, e.g., lecithin, cephalin, sphingomyjelin.

Phosphatidates—phospholipids minus the organic bases

Glycolipids—compounds of the fatty acids with a carbohydrate and containing nitrogen but no phosphoric acid, e.g., cerebrosides.

Sulfolipids—lipid molecules containing sulfuric acid radicles.

(Aminolipids, etc., not yet well characterized.)

Derivatives of Liqids

Fatty acids of various series.

Alcohols, including glycerol—mostly large molecular alcohols, found in nature combined with the fatty acid and which are soluble in the fat solvents-cholesterol ($C_{27}H_{45}OH$), myricyl alcohol ($C_{30}H_{61}OH$), cetyl alcohol ($C_{16}H_{33}OH$), etc. (The term *sterols* has often been applied to complex hydroaromatic secondary alcohols such as cholesterol and ergosterol.

3.3. Fats

Fats are glyceryl esters of fatty acids and on hydrolysis yield three molecules of fatty acids and are molecule of glycerol. e.g.

$$\underset{\substack{\text{Stearin} \\ \text{(glyceryl tristearater)}}}{C_3H_5(C_{18}H_{35}O_2)_3} + 3\,H_2O \rightarrow \underset{\text{Glycerol}}{C_3H_5(OH)_3} + \underset{\text{Stearic acid}}{3\,C_{18}H_{36}O_2}.$$

The above reaction is called *Saponification*.

The liquid fats are generally called *fatty oils* or *fixed oils*. They term fixed oil is used for them as the spot made by dropping a fatty oil an paper cannot be removed by drying nor by washing with water.

The fat can be separated from a food item by drying the food and extracting the food material with puse ether. However, generally the food fats are separated from the materials, in which they are present, by mechanical means such as churning of butter and pressing out of olive, cotton - seed, peanut or soybean oil. In both the cases the fat soluble substances remain dissolved in separated fats if not removed or destroyed by some subsequent refining process.

The separated forms of fat occurring as such in commerce are often called the "visible" fat supply in contradistinction from the fat contained in other foods such as meats, eggs, milk, or cheese.

In 1942-44 soybeans came into greatly increased prominence as a source of commercial food fat in the United States. Peanut oil has also been growing in prominence

The natural foods which contribute the largest amounts of fats to out diet are the animal products — meats and bowl, milk and milk product, eggs etc.

Fats are often added to foods during their preparation, either as shortening, as a method of transferring heat in frying, or for flavour and richness in preparing vegetables, puddings, etc. often lecithin is added as emulsifying agent, but fats are by far the most important additives among the lipids.

Structure of Fat

The ratio of carbon and hydrogen to oxygen in fat molecule is much more than in a carbohydrate. Far example *tristearin* (a fat found in beef) has 110 atoms of hydrogen to 6 atoms of oxygen.

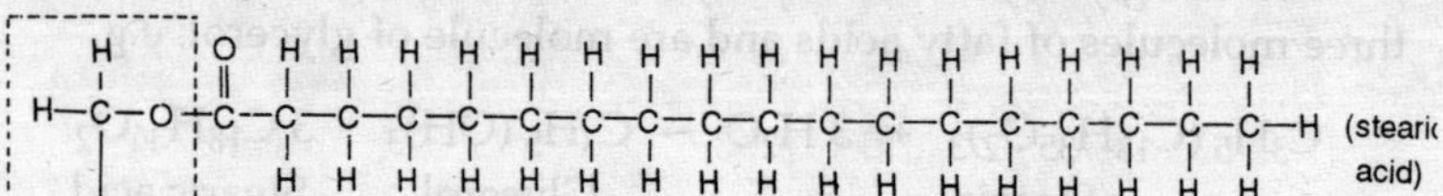

Fig. 3.1. The chemical formula of tristearin (a fat found in beef): $C_{57}H_{110}O_6$.

When a fat is burned in the body additional oxygen must be supplied by the cells to combine with all the carbon and hydrogen atoms, thus producing more heat. For this reason a gram of pure fat gives the body 9 Cal. of energy, whereas a gram of pure carbohydrate yields only 4 Cal.

The fats are triglycerides of fatty acids and the nature of fat depends on the kind of fatty acids, the length of the carbon chain of fatty acids and the degree of saturation or unsaturation of the fatty acids. Whether a glyceride will exist in liquid or solid state also depends upon the kind of fatty acid in its structure oil (liquid fat) contains more of unsaturated fatty acid that a solid fat. Oils are found in plants where as fats are of animal origin. The fats of animal differ from species to species. As a general rule we can say that fats in the more active parts of the animal organism have lower melting points and are more unsaturated and so they are more easily oxidised in comparison to those fats which are stored as fatty tissues.

Some Chemical substances, called as *antioxidants* help to delay to oxidation of "double-bond" linkages in a glyceride. They prolong the shelf life of a fat or oil. There are both natural and synthetic antioxidants. Vitamins C and E are examples of natural antioxidants; gallates and BHT (butylated hydroxytoluene) are examples of synthetic ones. Antioxidants apparently function in that they themselves are more easily oxidized than the glycerides they protect. "As a rule, it can be said that these substances have little effect on vegetable oils but a pronounced action on being added to animal oils and fats".

Before proceeding to hydrogenation of oils and fats we would like to know about- fatty acids.

3.4. Fatty Acids

They are the compounds of carbon, hydrogen and oxygen and are found in all simple and compound lipids. The simplest fatty acid is acetic acid (CH_3 COOH), the greater number of fatty acids belong to a few homologous series and can be represented by the general formula $c_n H_{2n} O_2$. Nearly all the fatty acids occurring in nature have even number of carbon atom. A few of the common fatty acids found in fats are butyric acid, Caprice acid, myristic acid, palmitic acid, stearic acid, oleic acid and linoleic acid.

Butyric acid, $CH_3 (CH_2)_2COOH$, found as glyceride to the extent of about 5 to 6 per cent in butter and in very small quantities in a few other fats.

Caproic acid, $CH_3 (CH_2)_4COOH$, is obtained from goat and cow butter and coconut fat.

Caprylic acid, $CH_3 (CH_2)_6COOH$, is obtained from coconut oil, goat and cow butter, and human fat.

Capric acid, $CH_3 (CH_2)_8COOH$, is obtained from coconut oil, goat and cow butter, and the fat of the spice bush.

Lauric acid, $CH_3 (CH_2)_{10}COOH$, occurs abundantly as glyceride in the fat of the seeds of the spice bush, and in smaller proportions in butter, coconut fat, palm oil, and some other vegetable oils.

Myristic acid, $CH_3 (CH_2)_{12}COOH$, is obtained from nutmeg butter, coconut oil, butter, lard, and many other fats, as well as from spermaceti and wool wax.

Palmitic acid, $CH_3 (CH_2)_{14}COOH$, occurs abundantly in a great variety of fats, both animal and vegetable, including many fatty oils, and also in several waxes, including spermaceti and beeswax.

Stearic acid, $CH_3 (CH_2)_{16}COOH$, is found in most fats, occurring more abundantly in the solid fats and especially in those having high melting points.

Butyric acid is a mobile liquid. It mixes in all proportions with water, alcohol, and ether; boiling without decomposition; and readily volatile with steam. With increasing molecular weight, the acids of this series regularly shows increasing boiling or melting points, and decreasing solubility and volatility. For ordinary temperatures the dividing line between liquids and solids falls at about caproic acid. Stearic acid is a crystalline solid, insoluble in water, and only moderately soluble in alcohol and ether.

The types of fatty acids found in foods are classified as short-chain (under 12 carbon atoms), long-chain (16 to 18 carbon atoms), and extra long-chain fatty acids (more than 20 carbon atoms), but in the average diet most of them are of the long-chain variety. Short-chain fatty acids are found in coconut oil, milk fat, and butterfat; the extra long-chain ones occur in fish oils and peanut oil (Table 3.1).

Table 3.1. Some of the Fatty Acids Found in Fats

Name	Number of Carbon Atoms	Classi-fication	Type	The food item in which they occur
Acetic	2	short	saturated	vinegar
Butyric	4	short	saturated	butter
Caproic	6	short	saturated	butter
Caprylic	8	short	saturated	coconut
Myristic	14	long	saturated	nutmeg and mace
palmitic	16	long	saturated	lard and palm oil
Stearic	18	long	saturated	beef tallow
Oleic	18	long	monounsaturated	olive oil
Linoleic	18	long	polyunsaturated	corn oil
Clupanadonic	22	extra long	polyunsaturated	fish oils

The fatty acids are also classified as saturated and unsaturated fatty acids.

Saturated Fatty Acids

Fatty acids such as stearic acids, contain as many hydrogen atoms as the carbon chain can hold and comprise about 40% of fatty acids contained in average diet. Most of these are concentrated in foods from animal sources. Chocolate and coconut (plant products) also contain appreciable quantities of fatty acids. In butter and cow milk the amount of stearic acid is about 12%. The palmitic acid in most animal fats in about 20-30 %.

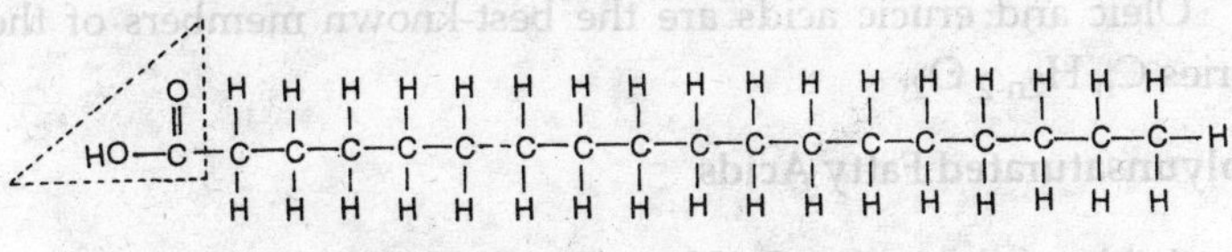

Fig. 3.2. Steric acid (safurated) $C_{18}H_{36}O_2$.

Unsaturated Fatty Acids

They are unsaturated compounds and each molecule contains one or more "double bond." They can take up halogen by addition to form a saturated compound; or, with a suitable catalyst, hydrogen may be added (hydrogenation). The relative number of double bonds can be measured analytically by determining the percentage of iodine which the fat or fatty acid will absorb. This is known as the *iodine number.* Thus pure oleic acid(mol. wt. 282) absorbs 2 atoms of iodine, giving an iodine number of 90; pure linoleic acid would absorb 4 atoms of iodine to the molecule, giving an iodine number about twice as great; and so on. These unsaturated acids have, much lower melting points than the saturated acids containing the same number of carbon atoms; and their fats are correspondingly softer. Such soft fats or fatty oils can be hardened to any desired consistency (up to that of stearin) by hydrogenations, which changes the unsaturated fatty acids radicles into the corresponding more saturated acid.

Monounsaturated Fatty Acids

The best example of this type is the long chain fatty acid (monounsaturated fatty acid), oleic acid which is found in appreciable amounts is most foods.

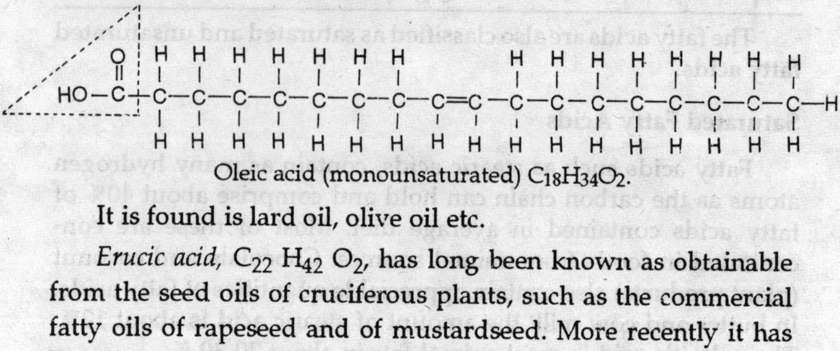

Oleic acid (monounsaturated) $C_{18}H_{34}O_2$.

It is found is lard oil, olive oil etc.

Erucic acid, $C_{22}H_{42}O_2$, has long been known as obtainable from the seed oils of cruciferous plants, such as the commercial fatty oils of rapeseed and of mustardseed. More recently it has been found also in marine animal oils (Hilditch).

Oleic and erucic acids are the best-known members of the series $C_nH_{2n-2}O_2$.

Polyunsaturated Fatty Acids

Acids of the series $C_nH_{2n-4}O_2$, $C_nH_{2n-6}O_2$ and $C_nH_{2n-8}O_2$ have now been found to occur as glycerides in many fats. *Linoleic acid,* $C_{18}H_{32}O_2$, and *linolenic acid,* $C_{18}H_{30}O_2$, take their names from having been first found in linseed oil; *arachidonic acid,* $C_{20}H_{32}O_2$, occurs in the lipids of the brain, liver, and other organs, and of

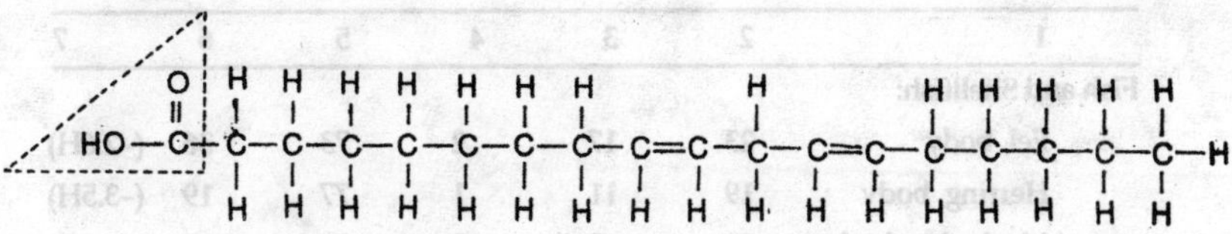

Linoleic acid (prolyunsaturated) $C_{18}H_{32}O_2$

egg yolks. These are but examples; probably many other fatty acids of these series may occur in natural fats.

Table 3.2. Fatty Acid Content of Food Fats (gram per 100 gm ether extract or crude fat)[1]

Food Fat or Oil	Saturated Fatty Acids Total[2]	Palmitic	Stearic	Unsaturated Fatty Acids Total[3]	Oleic	Linoleic
1	2	3	4	5	6	7
Animal Products						
Meats:						
Beef	48	28	19	47	44	2
Buffalo	66	34	28	30	24	1
Deer	63	24	34	32	24	3
Goat	57	26	24	37	33	2
Horse	30	24	5	60	30	6
Lamb	56	29	25	40	36	3
Luncheon meats	36	24	11	59	45	7
Pork:						
Back, outer layer	38	26	12	58	46	6
Bacon	32	21	9	63	48	9
Liver	34	13	18	61	27	5
Other cuts	36	21	13	59	42	9
Rabbit, domesticated	38	28	4	58	35	11
Milk Fat:						
Buffalo, Indian	62	29	15	33	26	1
Cow	55	25	12	39	33	3
Goat	62	27	8	33	25	5
Human	46	22	7	48	34	7
Poultry and Eggs:						
Chicken	32	24	7	64	38	20
Turkey	29	22	6	67	43	21
Chicken eggs	32	25	7	61	44	7

(Contd.)

1	2	3	4	5	6	7
Fish and Shellfish:						
Eel, body	23	17	2	73	36	(–2.6H)
Herring, body	19	11	1	77	19	(–3.5H)
Menhaden, body	24	15	3	71	15	3
Salmon, body	15	12	2	79	26	(–2.8H)
Tuna, body	25	18	3	70	25	(–3.2H)
Turtle	44	16	7	51	31	(–2.6H)
Separated Fats and Oils:						
Butter	55	25	12	39	33	3
Lard	38	31	7	57	46	10
Codfish liver	15	12	1	81	25	(–3.3H)
Halibut liver	17	13	Trace	72	31	—
Whale blubber	15	9	1	41	21	(–2.41H)
Plant Products						
Cereals and Grains:						
Cornmeal, white	11	8	1	82	34	44
Millet (Foxtail)	31	10	14	61	20	35
Cereals and Grains:						
Oats, rolled	22	13	4	74	32	41
Rice	17	12	2	74	39	35
Sorghum	12	7	5	81	37	44
Wheat flour, white	14	10	4	76	31	42
Wheat germ	15	11	4	77	23	48
Fruits and Vegetables Including Seeds:						
Avocado pulp	20	18	2	69	45	13
Cantaloupe seed	15	10	4	79	26	53
Chickpea	9	4	2	87	50	36
Chocolate	56	23	33	39	37	2
Olives	11	9	2	84	76	7
Pigeon pea	33	—	—	57	6	46
Pumpkinseed	17	9	8	78	37	41
Rapeseed	6	2	2	89	16	14
Sesame seed	14	8	4	80	38	42
Soybeans	20	11	7	75	16	52
Squash seed	18	12	6	77	35	42

(Contd.)

1	2	3	4	5	6	7
Watermelon seed	17	10	6	78	18	59
Nuts and Peanuts:						
Almond	8	7	1	87	67	20
Beechnut	8	5	3	87	54	31
Brazil nut	20	14	6	76	48	26
Cashew	17	6	11	78	70	7
Coconut	86	10	2	8	7	Trace
Filbert (Hazelnut)	5	2	2	91	54	16
Hickory	8	6	1	87	68	18
Peanut	22	11	4	72	43	29
Peanut butter	26	11	6	70	45	25
Pecan	7	6	1	84	63	20
Pistachio	10	8	2	85	65	19
Walnut, black	6	3	2	90	35	48
Walnut, English	7	5	2	89	15	62
Separated Fats and Oils:						
Cacao butter	56	23	33	39	37	2
Corn oil	10	8	2	84	28	53
Cottonseed oil	25	22	2	71	21	50
Margarine	26	21	3	70	57	9
Olive oil	11	9	2	84	76	7
Palm oil	45	39	4	49	40	8
Peanut oil	18	8	6	76	47	29
Separated Fats and Oils:						
Safflower oil	8	3	4	87	15	72
Sesame oil	14	8	4	80	38	42
Shortening (animal and vegetable)	43	27	12	53	41	11
Shortening (vegetable)	23	14	6	72	65	7
Soybean oil	15	9	6	80	20	52
Sunflower oil	12	6	5	83	20	63

1 To calculate fatty acids in foods, multiply amount (gm) of fat in food portion by value of each fatty acid. Trace is used to indicate values of 0.5 or less.

2 Includes other saturated fatty acids in addition to palmitic and stearic.

3 Includes other unsaturated fatty acids in addition to oleic and linoleic.

3.5. Hydrogenation of Fats and Oils

The oils from plants may be hardened to form solid glycerides or "soft" fats may be hardened to increase their melting points by the process of *Hydrogenation*. Previously the process of *non-selective hydrogenation* was used in which the oil was completely hydrogenated and then mixed with other glycerides to obtain a product of desired consistency. At present *selective hydrogenation* is alone in which partial hydrogenation is done to increase the firmness of glyceride without producing saturated fatty acids. In this polyunsaturated fatty acids get converted to monounsaturated fatty acids.

It has now been established that in man the blood cholesterol response to a dietary in take of partially hydrogenated vegetable fats and oils has been observed to be equivalent to the response from unhydrogenated vegetable oils.

3.6. Functions of Fats and Oils

They are the source of energy and of essential fatty acids in the diet. In addition fat deposits in the body serve as insulation and provide protective cushion for the organs.

The chief contribution of fats and other lipids to diet in their energy value (approximately a calories / g). Moreover, the greatest supply of reserve energy in animals and man is found in the fat stores of the body.

Essential fatty acid are those fatty acids which man needs for good health and which the body cannot produce. (e.g. linoleic acid, linolenic acid arachidonic acid). It has now been proved that arachidonic acid can be formed in the body from linoleic acid. Linolenic acid has also been found to have a less important function than lenoleic acid.

In the animal organism linoleic acid plays an essential role in reproduction and lactation. It also acts as a protective agent against radiation effects and also prevents the excess loss of water from the body by preventing the development of the permeability of shin capillaries.

Though not much is human about the essential fatty acid requirements of a man but it has been found that it is sufficient if a child is given the linoleic acid that provides him about 4 % of total calories.

A low fat diet infant shows a tendency towards skin disorder and a high fat in take has a positive correlation with blood cholesterol level.

Another important function performed by fats is to support and provide cushion to the viscera and certain organs of body such as kidneys.

Fats are also solvents for the fat soluble vitamins that are always naturally introduced into the diet in the fatty portion of the food. The fat soluble vitamins are vitamins A, D, E and K and the provitamins A, the carotenes. All of these vitamins are important to optimum health.

3.7. The Phospholipids and Sterols

Phosphatidic acids are compounds containing glycerol, two fatty acids and a phosphate group and they give rise to triglycerides or to phospholipids

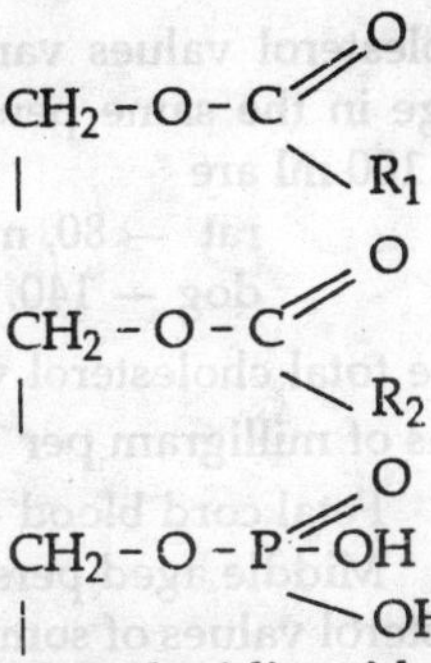

phosphatidic acid

The phospholipids differ chiefly in the specific compound attached to the phosphate group of the phosphatidic core. Some of the important phospholipids are *Lecithins, Cephalins* etc.

Phospholipids are widely distributed in living cells and are found in every living cell. They are essential to the structure and function of the cell. They aid in the transport of fatty acids in the body.

In general there is a larger proportion of unsatruation in fatty acids of the phosphatids than in those of "neutral" or "depot" fats (the glycerides such as those of adipose tissue). They are active intermediates in the biosynthesis of other lipid compounds and they do not accumulate in tissues in significant amounts.

Phospholipids have the useful property of attracting both water soluble and fat soluble substance due to the hydrophilic phosphoryl group and hydrophobic fatty acid in the molecule. In combination with proteins, they are the constituents of cell membranes and membranes of subcellular particles where they serve as a liaison between fat solùble and water soluble materials that must penetrate the membrane and interact once they have gained entry. In this structural role phospholipids are not generally available as an energy source. Even a starved animal will retain the phospholipid necessary to maintain the integrity of tissue cells.

Sterols : These are the alcohol-like steroids and they do not contain carbonyl or carboxy groups common to other steroids.

The most common sterol in animal tissues is *Cholesterol* which occurs in free form or combined in esters formation with fatty acids. Cholesterol is present in *only* animals though many other sterols are found in plant tissues. Some but not all sterols are among the vitamin D.

Blood cholesterol values vary from species to species and varies with age in the same person. The average values per in milligram per 100 ml are

rat — 80, monkey — 120
dog — 140, man — 220

In man the total cholesterol values changes with age. These values in terms of milligram per 100 ml are as follows.

Fetal cord blood – 65, young adult – 190
Middle aged person – 245.

The cholesterol values of some items used in food as given in Table 3.3.

Table 3.3
Chdesterol Content of Foods

Food	*Cholesterol per 100 gm Edible Portion, in mg*	*Food*	*Cholesterol per 100 gm Edible Portion, in mg*
Beef, raw	70	Kidney, raw	375
Butter	250	Lamb, raw	70
Cheese:		Lard and other	
Cheddar	100	animal fat	95
cottage, creamed	15	Liver, raw	300
cream	120	Lobster	200
other (25 to 30% fat)	85	Margarine:	
Cheese spread	65	all vegetable fat	0
Chicken, raw	60	two-thirds animal	

(*Contd.*)

Crabmeat	125	fat, one-third	
Egg, whole	550	vegetable fat	65
Egg, white	0	Milk:	
Egg yolk:		fluid, whole	11
fresh	1500	dried, whole	85
frozen	1280	fluid, skin	3
dried	2950	Mutton	65
Fish, steak or fillet	70	Pork	70
Heart, raw	150	Shrimp	125
Ice cream	45	Veal	90

3.8. Relationship of Dietary Fat to Artherosclerosis

Artheroclerosis is a diseases in which the wales of arteries thicken owing to deposits of fats and mineral salts. This condition makes a person more susceptible to heart attacks and heart strokes. *Cholesterol* has achieved a certain amount of notoriety as a factor in the development of artheroclerosis and heart disease. A high incidence of heart disease is most often associated with high level of serum cholesterol.

The influence of cholesterol in the diet on the blood level of this constituents is uncertain. It has non been found that the body could synthesize cholesterol at the rate of 2-3g per day and the average diet provides only about 0.5g per day so the role of dietary cholesterol is not of much consequence. However, Those fats in which cholesterol is most soluble do tend to elevate cholesterol level in blood.

Some other factors, than nutrients, also influence the cholesterol level of the blood. Exercise is are such factor. The other one is number of times a diet is taken in a day.

Although no direct relationship between diet or serum lipid concentration and the cause of atherosclerosis has been proven yet, the regulation of dietary fat is now a suggested medical procedure in the treatment of certain diseases. The Council of Foods and Nutrition of the American Medical Association has recommended to the medical profession that the diet's total fat content in gall bladder disease, certain types of malabsorption, and hypertriglyceridemia be restricted, as well as an increase of dietary polyunsaturated fats in hypercholesteremia.

4

The Proteins and the Amino-Acids

4.1. Introduction

Proteins are a large number of different but related nitrogenous organic compounds which are so prominent among the constituents of the tissues and in the cost of food that they may still be accorded some degree of preeminence in a study of the chemistry of food and nutrition.

The word protein, derived from the Greek language means "to come first. Gerardus Mulder" the famous Dutch chemist (1802-1880), proposed use of the term because he believed that proteins were "unquestionably the most important of all known substances in the organic kingdom".

Proteins are essential constituents of both plant and animal cells.

While plants are able to utilize inorganic sources of nitrogen such as ammonia, nitrates etc., man and other higher animals are for the most part dependent on a source of amino acids to build their body proteins.

In man synthesis of many proteins that make up body tissues require the presence of amino acids. About 20 amino acids are in the body proteins. All of the 20 amino acids are not required in the diet as the man is capable of synthesizing all of the amino acids except 8 (leucine, isoleucine, lysine, valine thireonine, tryptophan, phenylalanine and methionine). However, some sources of nitrogen in the amino form must be available. The amino group from other amino acid enters the nitrogen pool and can be used for the synthesis of any amino acid whose carbon skeleton can be made Man's food must supply sufficient amino acids for the purpose of building proteins.

4.2. Proteins

Protein is one of the most abundant components in the body (next only to water), though major protion of protein is located in muscle tissue, it is widely distributed in blood, bones, teeth and other soft tissues.

Protein contains the elements carbon hydrogen, oxygen and nitrogen. The other elements present are sulphur, phosphorus, iron, iodine and cobalt.

Generally speaking, the proteins of different kinds of tissues and even of corresponding tissues of different species are not identical substances. However, with in a species the same proteins are synthesized by all members. This is called *protein specificity.*

4.3. Classification of Proteins

The classification of proteins given here is in accordance with the recommendations made by the American Physiological Society and the American Society of Biological chemists.

I. Simple Proteins

Protein substances which yield only amino acids or their derivatives on complete hydrolysis. Examples are albumen of egg, zein of corn, keratin of hair and globin of haemoglobin etc,

(a) *Albumins* : Simple proteins soluble in pure water and coagulable by heat. Examples: egg albumin, serum albumin (blood), leucosin (wheat), legumelin (peas).

(b) *Globulins* : Simple proteins insoluble in water, but soluble in neutral salt solutions. Examples : muscle globulin, serum globulin (blood), edestin (wheat, hemp seed, and other seeds), phaseolin (beans), legumin (beans and peas), vignin (cow peas), tuberin (potato), amandin (almonds), excelsin (Brazil nuts), arachin and conarachin (peanuts).

(c) *Glutelins* : Simple proteins insoluble in all neutral solvents, but readily soluble in very dilute acids and alkalies. The best known and most important member of this group is the glutenin of wheat.

(d) *Alcohol soluble proteins (prolamins)* : Simple proteins soluble in relatively strong alcohol (70-80 per cent) but insoluble in water, absolute alcohol, and other neutral solvents. Examples: gliadin (wheat), zein (maize), hordein (barley), kafirin (kafircorn).

(e) *Albuminoids* : These are simple proteins characteristic of the skeletal structures of animals (so they are also known as scleroproteins) and also of the external protective tissues, such as the skin, hair, etc. Example: collagen, which when boiled with water yields gelatin.

(f) *Histones* : Soluble in water, and insoluble in very dilute ammonia, and in the absence of ammonium salts insoluble even in an excess of ammonia. They yield precipitates with solutions of other proteins and a coagulum an heating which is easily soluble in very dilute acids. When hydrolysed they yield various amino acids, among which the basic ones predominate. The only members of this group which have any considerable importance as food are the thymus histone and the globin of hemoglobin.

(g) *Protamins* : These are simpler substances and are soluble in water, not coagulable by heat, possess strong basic properties, and on hydrolysis yield a few amino acids, among which the basic amino acids greatly predominate. They are of no importance as food.

II. Conjugated Proteins or Compound Proteins

Substances which contain the protein molecule united to some other non-protein molecule or molecules or with a metal. Examples are haemoglobin (protein + heme) of blood, Casein (protein + phosphoric acid) of milk, mucin (protein + carbohydrate) of saliva and lipo-protein (protein + lipid) in blood plasma.

(*a*) *Nucleoproteins* : Compounds of one or more protein molecules with nucleic acid. Examples of the nucleic acids thus found united with proteins are thymo-nucleic acid (thymus gland), triticonucleic acid (wheat germ).

(*b*) *Glycoproteins* : Compounds of the protein molecule with a substance or substances containing a carbohydrate group other than a nucleic acid. Example: mucins.

(*c*) *Phosphoproteins* : Compounds in which the phosphorus is in organic union with the protein molecule otherwise than in a nucleic acid or lecithin. Examples: caseinogen (milk), ovovitellin (egg yolk).

(*d*) *Hemoglobins* : Compounds of the protein molecule with hematin or some similar substance. Examples: hemoglobin of blood. (The redness of meat is also due chiefly to hemoglobin.)

(*e*) *Lecithoproteins* : Compounds of the protein molecule with lecithins or related substances.

III. Derived Proteins

Products formed from the partial breakdown of proteins by the action of heat and other physical forces, or by hydrolytic agents. Examples are peptones, polypeptides, and peptides which are mixtures of amino acids with decreasing numbers of amino acids in the chain length.

Primary protein derivatives : Derivatives of the protein molecule that are apparently formed through hydrolytic changes which involve only slight changes.

(*a*) *Proteans* : Insoluble products that is obtained from the incipient action of water, very dilute acids, or enzymes. Examples: casein (curdled milk), fibrin (coagulated blood).

(*b*) *Metaproteins* : Products of the further action of acids and alkalies whereby the molecule is sufficiently changed to form proteins soluble in very weak acids and alkalies, but insoluble in neutral solvents. This group includes the substances that are known as "acid proteins," "acid albumins," "syntonin," "alkali proteins," "alkali albumins," and "albuminates."

IV. Coagulated Proteins

Insoluble products obtained from (1) the action of heat on protein solutions, or (2) the action of alcohol on the protein. Example: cooked egg albumin, or egg albumin precipitated by means of alcohol.

Secondary protein derivatives : Products obtained by the further hydrolytic cleavage of the protein molecule.

(*a*) *Proteoses* : Soluble in water, not coagulable by heat, precipitated by saturating their solutions with ammonium sulfate or zinc sulfate. The products commercially called "peptones" made up of largely of proteoses.

(*b*) *Peptones* : Soluble in water, not coagulable by heat, and not precipitated by saturating their solutions with ammonium sulfate or zinc sulfate. These represent a further stage of cleavage than the proteoses. (The term "peptone" was formerly used for all digestion products not coagulated by boiling and is still popularly used in the same sense.)

(*c*) *Peptides* : Definitely characterized combinations of two or more amino acids. An anhydride of two amino acid radicles is a "di-peptide"; one having three amino acid radicles is a "tri-peptide"; etc. Peptides are obtained from the further hydrolytic cleavage of the peptones. Many peptides have also been made in the laboratory by the linking together of amino acids.

Substances simpler that the peptones but containing several amino acid radicles are known as "poly-peptides".

4.4. Chemical Nature and Physical Properties of Proteins

Generally speaking, the proteins of different kinds of tissue, and even of the corresponding tissues of different species, are not identical substances. The total number of different proteins found in nature must therefore be very great. The natural proteins are found to be very complex substances and the chemical structure of a none of these typical natural protein has been *fully* determined. It has, however, been shown that the typical proteins are essentially anhydrides of the amino acids:

Amino acids are considered as "building stavas" of protein. An amino acid is a compound that contains an amino ($-NH_2$) group and a carboxylic acid ($-$ COOH) group e.g glycine, alanime etc

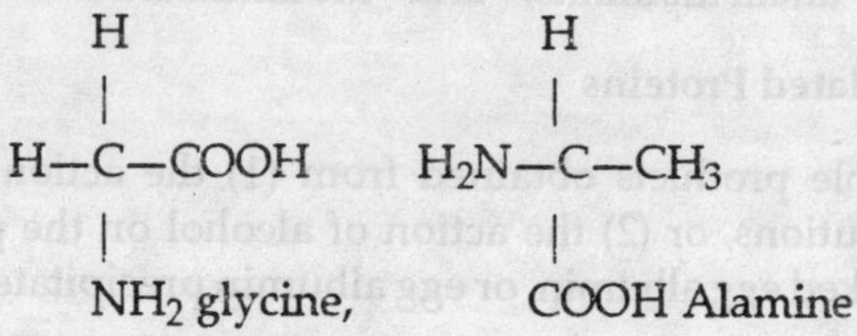

Chemical structures of some more amino acids are as follows.

Monoamino-monocarboxylic acids

Glycine, amino- acetic acid, $CH_2(NH_2) \cdot COOH$

Alanine, α-amino-propionic acid, $CH_3 \cdot CH(NH_2) \cdot COOH$

Valine, α-amino-β-methyl-n-butyric acid,

$$(CH_3)_2 : CH \cdot CH(NH_2) \cdot COOH$$

Leucine, α-amino-γ-methyl, *n*-valeric acid,

$$(CH_3)_2 : CH \cdot CH_2 \cdot CH(NH_2) \cdot COOH$$

Isoleucine, α-amino-β-methyl-n-valeric acid,

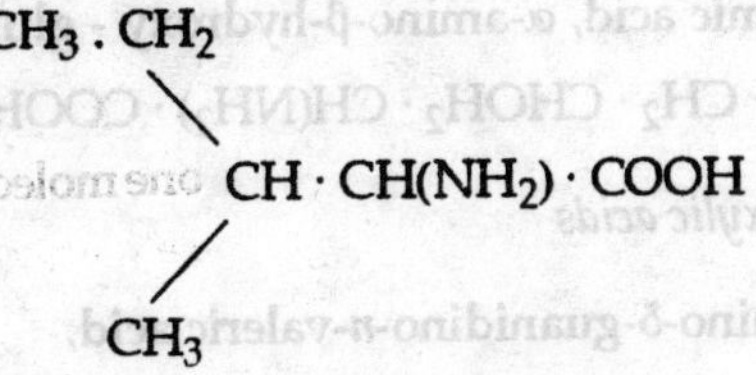

Noreucine, α-amino -n-caproic acid,

$$CH_3 \cdot CH_2 \cdot CH_2 \cdot CH_2 \cdot CH(NH_2) \cdot COOH$$

Phenylalanine, α-amino-β-phenyl-propionic acid,

$$C_6H_5CH_2 \cdot CH(NH_2) \cdot COOH$$

Tyrosine, α-amino-β-para-hydroxphenyl-propionic acid,

$$C_6H_4(OH) \cdot CH_2\ CH(NH_2) \cdot COOH$$

Serine, α-amino-β-hydroxy-propionic acid,

$$CH_2(OH) \cdot CH(NH_2) \cdot COOH$$

Threonine a α-amino-β-hydroxy-*n*-butyric acid,

$$CH_3 \cdot CH(OH) \cdot CH(NH_2) \cdot COOH$$

Cystine (dicysteine), or di-(α-amino-β-thio- propionic acid),

$$\begin{array}{l} S \cdot CH_2.\ CH(NH_2) \cdot COOH \\ | \\ S \cdot CH_2.\ CH(NH_2) \cdot COOH \end{array}$$

Methionine, α-amino-γ-methylthio-*n*-nityric acid,

$$CH_3 \cdot S \cdot CH_2, CH_2 \cdot CH(NH_2) \cdot COOH$$

Monoamino-dicarboxylic acids

Aspartic acid, amino-succinic acid,

$$COOH \cdot CH_2 \cdot CH(NH_2) \cdot COOH$$

Glutamic (glutaminic) acid, α-amino-glutaric acid,

$$COOH \cdot CH_2 \cdot CH_2 \cdot CH(NH_2) \cdot COOH$$

Hudroxyglutamic acid, α-amino-β-hydroxy - glutaric acid,

$$COOH \cdot CH_2 \cdot CHOH_2 \cdot CH(NH_2) \cdot COOH$$

Diamino-monocarboxylic acids

Arginine, α-amino-δ-guanidino-*n*-valeric acid,

NH

..

$$(H_2N)\ C \cdot NH \cdot CH_2 \cdot CH_2 \cdot CH_2 \cdot CH\ (NH_2) \cdot COOH$$

Lysine, α, ∈, diamino-*n*-caproic acid,

$$CH_2\ (NH_2) \cdot CH_2 \cdot CH_2 \cdot CH_2 \cdot CH\ (NH_2) \cdot COOH$$

Heterocyclic amino acids

Histidine, α-amino-β-imidazole propionic acid,

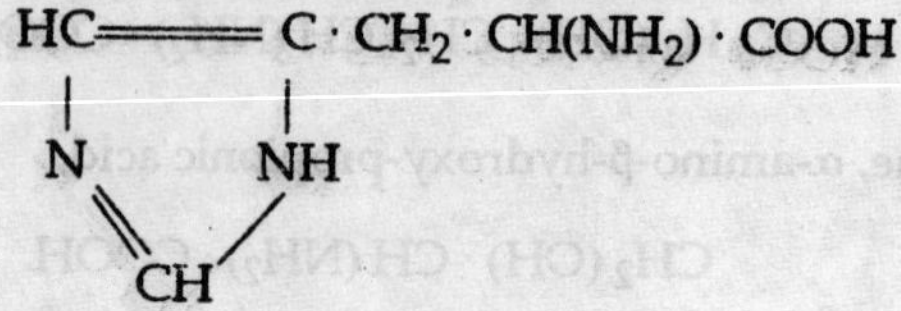

Proline, α-pyrrolidine-carbxylic acid,

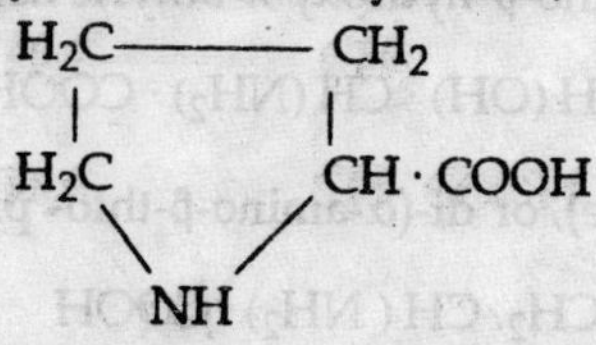

Hydroxproline, γ-hydroxy-α-pyrrolidine-carboxylic acid,

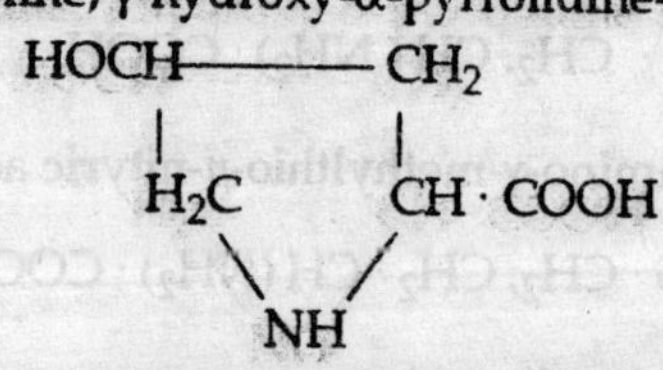

Tryptophane, α-amino-β-indole-propionic acid,

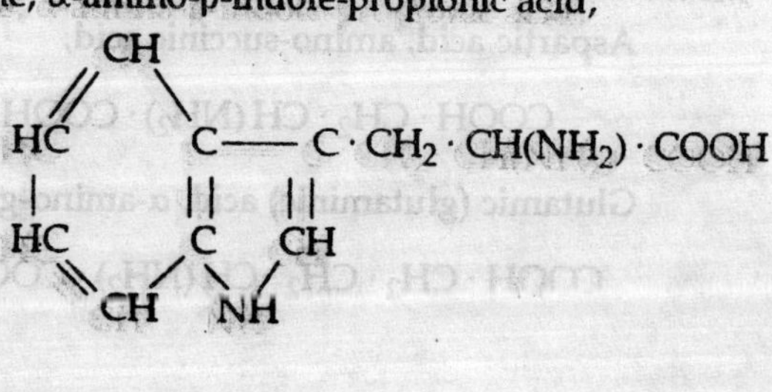

Carbohydrate radicle found in most of the proteins is also considered as a component of protein molecule. In some proteins a carbohydrate complex made up of two molecules of hexose and one molecule of hexosamine are found. The hexoses generally present are mannose, galactose, or a mixture of mannose and galactose.

Most of the proteins are α-amino proteins. The exception to this being proline and hydroxyproline and in them the α-amino group is condensed with the delta - carbon.

The linkage of amino acid radicles in the protein molecule is chiefly through carboxyl group of one amino acid reacting with the amino group of another. Thus two molecules of glycine combined by elimination of one molecule of water, yield glycylglycine.

$$H_2N - CH_2 - C = O$$

$$H'N - CH_2\ COOH$$

It is the simplest group of an hydrides of amino acids called *peptides. Dipeptides* contain two amino acid radicles and tripeptides three and so on.

Amino acids are white crystalline substances, each with an individual microscopic structure. They differ in taste; some are sweet (glycine, alanine and serine), some are tasteless (tryptophan and leucine), others are bitter (arginine).

Molecular Weights of Proteins

Two molecular weight of protein of Egg albumin is about 34500 and the molecular weights of many other typical proteins are about 1, 2, 3, or 6 times the molecular weight of egg albumin.

4.5. Functions of Protein

1. To Provide Amino Acids to Body

An important function of dietary protein is the provision of amino acids for the body to build new tissue and to maintain the tissue already formed.

2. Formation of other Nitrogen Containing Substances

In addition, amino acids are used to form nitrogen-containing substances essential to body functions, such as the enzymes, antibodies and hormones.

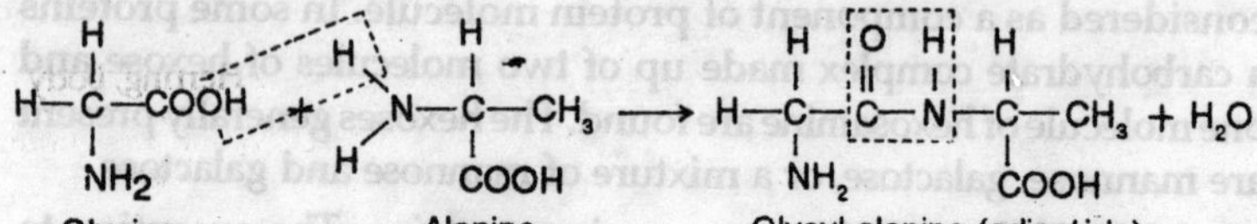

Fig. 4.1. Chemical formulas of two amino acids, glycine and alanine, showing the formation of a dipeptide by the peptide linkage.

3. Proteins serves also in certain body regulating capacities and provides energy.

Body Regulating Substance

Movement of fluid : Protein is one of the factors that contributes to the control of fluid movement in and out of cells and movement to and from the blood stream. The large size of the protein molecule avoids its passage through membranes, whereas water and materials in solution pass readily. Fluids move from a medium of lesser concentration to one of greater concentration. The process (osmosis) is one of the means the body has of maintaining normal composition of the blood and other body fluids.

Maintenance of normal reaction in the tissues : There are several mechanisms for maintaining a normal balance between acidic and basic substances in the body. Blood proteins help to maintain the normal, slightly alkaline reaction of the blood by the buffering action of protein in the blood plasma and the action of hemoglobin in the red cells. Hemoglobin, a conjugated protein, carries CO_2 to the lungs to be eliminated as a gas. If CO_2 was not eliminated it would dissolve in water and form carbonic acid. Thus hemoglobin and the lungs work together in the regulation of the acid-base balance of the blood and extracellular fluid.

Source of Energy

One gram of protein supplies approximately 4 Cal. In the average American diet 10 to 15 per cent of the energy value of the diet comes from protein sources. The extent protein is used for energy depends on the amount of carbohydrate and fat in the diet as well as the total intake of protein. Even though protein is primarily considered a body-building and body- regulation substance, the function of providing energy takes precedence when the carbohydrate and fat in the diet furnish insufficient Calories. There are several pathways that this fraction may take; it may be oxidized directly; it may be converted to either carbohydrate or fat; or it may be changed back to certain amino acids (the nonessential amino acids) by adding an available amino group, a process by which amino acids can be synthesized in the body. As for the nitrogen removed from the protein, most of it is eliminated as waste by way of the kidney.

4.6. The Nutritional Value of Proteins

In most of the cases studied it has been found that the nutrition values of food proteins depend essentially upon the kinds of amino acids radicles which they contain and the quantitative proportion of each.

On the basis of their nutritive quality the proteins has been classified as (*i*) complete proteins and (*ii*) partially complete or incomplete proteins.

Complete proteins maintain life and provide for normal growth of the young when used as the only protein in the diet of experimental animals. As a general rule, the proteins of animal source are complete including those of meat, fish, fowl, eggs and milk; gelatin is an exception. Some proteins in legumes, grains, and nuts are complete such as glycinin of soybeans, glutenin of wheat, glutelin of corn, and excelsin in Brazil nuts.

Partially complete or *incomplete proteins* maintain life but fail to support normal growth. Examples include gliadin of wheat, hordein of barley, and prolamin of rye.

Incomplete proteins neither maintain life nor support growth. Most vegetable proteins are incomplete; the glycinin of soybeans is an exception. The zein of corn and the animal protein gelatin are incomplete.

Though all amino acids which are essential to the structure of body proteins are in this sense nutritionally essential substances; but the term *nutritionally essential* when used generally refers to the fact that the substance in question *must be fed* (i.e. furnished by nutrient constituent.

On the bases of experimental studies it has been found that there are ten amino acids which are needed in food in take and the body cannot synthesize them at the rate at which they are needed for growth. These are called "essential" or "indispensable" amino acids. These are given in Table 4.1

Table 4.1. Amino Acids Essential for Growth in the Young Rat, Growth in Children, and for Maintenance in Adult Men

Amino Acids	*Essential for Growth in Young Rats*	*Essential for Growth in Children*	*Essential for Maintenance in Young Men*
Arginine	x		
Histidine	x	x	
Isolencine	x	x	x
Leucine	x	x	x
Lysine	x	x	x
Methionine	x	x	x
Phenylalanine	x	x	x
Threonine	x	x	x
Tyrptophan	x	x	x
Valine	x	x	x

Those amino acids which are not needed in the diet, as they can be synthesized by the body at the rate needed by the body, are called "Non - essential" or "dispensable" amino acids.

From the Table 4.1 it is evident that Eight amino acids are essential in young men and nine amino acids are essentials in case of adults (human beings).

From this it may appear that exchange of atoms or radicles may supply some of the acids for the slow turn over of adult maintenance but not for relatively rapid retention involved in the upbuilding of new tissues in the normally growing young animals.

It must be emphasized here that the non - essential amino acids are in no may less important than essential amino acids for growth, development etc. of the body. Their importance can be guessed from the fact that they comprise 40% or more of tissue protein. For a normal growth essential : non-essential amino acids is about 4:1.

The nutritive value of protein also depends upon its *digestibility.*

Animal proteins are the most available for absorption and the proteins from dried legumes are least available because of less complete digestion.

The digestibility of protein depends upon its fibre content. It also depends upon the fibre content in the remainder of diet. The table 4.2 lists the digestibility of some proteins.

Table 4.2. Average Digestibility of Proteins from Different Food Groups

Food Group	*Coefficients of Availability, per cent*
Animal foods	97
Cereals	85
Fruits	85
Vegetables	83
Legumes, dried	78

The Requirements of Proteins and Amino Acids

When the intake and outgo of nitrogen are approximately the same, the individual is said to be in *nitrogen equilibrium*.

The *minimum nitrogen* intake that will allow the state of nitrogen equilibrium is considered *minimum nitrogen (proteins) requirement.*

To convert nitrogen values of food (determined by finding the nitrogen content of food) to protein it is multiplied by 6.25 because an average food proteins are 16% nitrogen.

The nitrogen balance of the body depends upon the following factors :

(*i*) The physiological state of the individual.

(*ii*) Adequacy of energy intake from carbohydrates and fats.

(*iii*) The capacity to adjust to level of intake.

Recommended Allowance for Proteins

For an adult (18 - 35 years) about 10 - 12% of total calories from proteins in diet are considered adequate. The needs for infancy, childhood, during pregnancy and lactation are more. More proteins are needed under conditions of stress. As opposed to general belief we do not need any more proteins during body exercises.

Increased Need for Protein Under Conditions of Stress

After surgery or injury, during a wasting illness, or while recovering from extensive burns, excessive loss of nitrogen from the body occurs. It is generally felt that these losses should be replaced through a liberal in take of protein.

Table 4.3. The Effect of Extremely Low Protein Intake on Nitrogen Excretion

		Average Daily Excretion, gm	
Days on Diet	*Average Daily Nitrogen Intake, gm*	*Urine*	*Feces*
7	Unrestricted diet	12.03	1.03
6	0.27	4.85	0.85
7	0.77	3.55	0.73
8	0.94	2.21	0.83
1	0.32	1.41	0.89
2	Unrestricted diet	9.21	—

Table 4.4. Influence of Work on Nitrogen Excretion

		Food/Day		
Activity	*Period, Days*	*Nitrogen, gm*	*Energy, Cal*	*Nitrogen Excreted, Daily Average, gm*
Bed rest	6	5.9	2300	4.77
Light exercise	5	6.0	3000	4.40
Heavy exercise	4	5.9	3200	3.94

Influence of Exercise on Protein Need

Though unexpected but it is a fact that exercise does not increase the protein need. If the caloric intake is sufficient to cover the increased energy requirement during exercise, then no additional protein is needed. It is quite logical because during exercise glycogen, not protein, is the ultimate constituent used up in muscle contraction. The data in Table 4.4 are taken from an early experiment in which a subject was maintained on the same nitrogen intake with adjustment in energy intake to take care of different degrees of exercise. No increase in the excretion of nitrogen resulted with exercise, reflecting no additional need for protein.

For normal persons the minimal requirement of proteins intake is about 0.6 g/kg of the body weight for maintenance of nitrogen equilibrium and the recommended daily intake is 1.0g/kg of the body weight.

Recent studies have confirmed that it is possible to maintain nitrogen equilibrium of body with intake of 0.55g/kg (instead of 0.6g/kg) even if the main source of protein in diet are cereals. The quantity may vary between 0.43 - 0.57g/kg with cereals, fruits and vegetables providing the proteins. If one third of the diet is replaced by protein of animal source it is possible to maintain equilibrium at an intake of only 0.39g/kg.

4.7. The FAO Reference Protein

The protein requirements were reported by a committee of FAO in 1957. For this the committee used a hypothetical protein referred as "reference protein" which was similar to proteins found in milk, egg and meat. A comparison of this 'reference protein' to the other three proteins in given in Table 4.5.

Table 4.5. Essential Amino Acids in Provisional Pattern and Milk and Egg Proteins

	Amino Acids per 100 gm Protein			
Amino Acids	*Provisional Pattern*	*Cow's Milk*	*Human Milk*	*Egg*
Isoleucine	4.2	6.4	6.4	6.8
Leucine	4.8	9.9	8.9	9.0
Lysine	4.2	7.8	6.3	6.3
Phenylalanine	2.8	4.9	4.6	6.0
Tyrosine	2.8	5.1	5.5	4.4
Methionine	2.2	2.4	2.2	3.1
Threonine	2.8	4.6	4.6	5.0
Tryptophan	1.4	1.4	1.6	1.7
Valine	4.2	6.9	6.6	7.4

According to this FAO committee report the average minimum requirement for adults for the "reference protein" is 0.35g/kg of body weight.

If was also suggested that the provisional pattern of amino acids can be used in appraising the protein (amino acids) value of diets and for indicating appropriate methods of supplementing diets deficient in protein (amino acids).

The minimum amounts of essential amino acids needed by adults are given in Table 4.6.

Table 4.6. Minimum Amounts of Essential Amino Acids Required Daily for Maintenance of Nitrogen Equilibrium in Adults

Essential Amino Acid	*Women, gm*	*Men, gm*
Isoleucine	0.45	0.70
Leucine	0.62	1.10
Lysine	0.50	0.80
Methionine	0.29	1.10
Phenylalanine	0.22	1.10
Threonine	0.31	0.50
Tryptophan	0.16	0.25
Valine	0.65	0.80

4.8. Protein Deficiency

Insufficient protein in the diet may result in stunted growth of the individual. If the limitation is severe and prolonged, the protein content of the blood may be reduced below normal (hypoproteinemia).

Four syndromes that are associated with protein deficiency in the human as described by the Food and Nutrition Boards are hunger edema, pellagra, kwashiorkar, and nutritional liver disease. Only nutritional liver disease is of consequence today. This disease is often seen in the alcoholic whose diet is low in essential nutrients, including protein; less frequently it occurs in individuals who are losing or destroying proteins at an abnormal rate or who are failing to synthesize adequate protein. The simplest form of nutritional liver disease is characterized by an enlarged fatty liver, which may be cured by eating an adequate diet.

Hunger edema was observed due to mass semi-starvation of civilians and in prison comps during World War II. The most prominent manifestation of hunger edema is the excessive retention of fluid in body cells and for it protein deficiency is only one of the factors.

A severe deficiency disease, *kwashiorkor,* found among the children of Africa and parts of Central and South America, is caused by a shortage in total amount of protein and also a shortage of protein of good quality. This disease is most prevalent in populations whose protein supply is chiefly of vegetable origin. If the diet is inadequate in protein, it is most certain to be so in other nutrients; for that reason the condition has been described as a "multiple-deficiency syndrome." Children between the ages of 1 and 4 are most commonly afflicted, although sporadic cases do occur among older children.

The children suffering with kwashiorkor manifest certain characteristic symptoms: they are stunted in growth; the skin shows hyperpigmentation and is frequently ulcerated; the children are apathetic showing marked lassitude, but at the same time are irritable and restless; the digestive system is impaired by continuous diarrhea; the children have poor appetites; anemia is always present; the incidence of dental caries is high; and the muscles are underdeveloped and lacking in tone.

Though the primary cause of kwashiorkor is protein deficiency but it occurs to varying degrees in conjunction with *calorie deficiency*. For this reason the present trend is to speak of protein - calorie malnutrition rather than kwashiorkor or marasums (another disease due to protein deficiency).

Since kwashiorkor develops when mother steps feeding the babies with breast milk and after weaning from protein rich breast-milk, the child from a poorer family is given a diet consisting mainly of carbohydrates, having a low protein content. The term 'kwashiorkor' mean 'rejected child' or 'neglected child'.

It can be prevented or cured by giving the child a sufficient quantity of protein rich diet as

(*a*) a combination of wheat, gram, pea-nuts, soyabean and jaggery;

(*b*) a diet with animal proteins like mutton, chicken and fish.

Marasums can be cured by giving the child adequate amount of diet containing proteins as well as carbohydrates and fats. In the absence of mother's milk, pure cow's milk may be given to the child.

In Central America after a good a discussion of preventive measures for the disease resulted in the following suggestions: that varieties of maize higher in mithionine and tryptophan content be developed; that the production of certain protein-producing plants now being consumed, such as beans, be increased; and that the use of soybean milk be promoted to substitute for milk unavailable in those areas.

4.9. Food Sources and Supply of Proteins and Amino Acids

Although protein is widely distributed in nature, few foods provide highly concentrated amounts (Table 4.7). Cheese, eggs, fish, meats, nuts, and poultry are the sources with a range of 12 to 29 per cent. Cereal grains are also protein contributors to the diet. Fruits and vegetables are low-protein foods. Those containing no protein are the sugars and sirups and the pure fats and oils.

Animal foods have protein high in nutritive quality and quantities. Soybeans and some nuts, such as Brazil and almonds, contain protein of good quality, and most cereals provide a limited amount.

Moreover plants are also fundamental to the production of animal proteins for human consumption. Nature has equipped plants with the capacity to take nitrogen available in the soil for the synthesis of amino acids and protein. Ruminant animals consume the proteins in plants and are able to use them as a source of nitrogen for the synthesis of their tissue proteins.

Table 4.7. Protein Values of Some Typical Foods

Food	*Measure*	*Protein, gm*
Chicken, breast	2.7 oz	25.0
Tuna fish	3 oz	24.0
Beef, round	3 oz	24.0
Lamb, leg	3 oz	22.0
pork loin	3 oz	20.0
Milk, whole	1 c	9.0
Beans, red kidney	$\frac{1}{2}$ c	7.5
Çheese, process	1 oz	7.0
Egg	1 med	6.0
Lima beans, immature	$\frac{1}{2}$ c	6.0
Bacon	2 sl	5.0
Peanut butter	1 tbsp	4.0
Ice cream	$\frac{1}{8}$ qt	3.0
Potato	1 med	3.0
Oatmeal	$\frac{1}{2}$ c	2.5
Broccoli	$\frac{1}{2}$ c	2.5
Bread, whole wheat	1 sl	2.0
Green beans	$\frac{1}{2}$ cl	1.0
Lettuce, head	$\frac{1}{2}$ c	0.6
Orange juice	4 oz	0.5

To get enough proteins are must include certain types of foods in his diet every day. In Table 4.8 are listed some items of food according to various lost levels, which provide sufficient proteins to an individuals need.

Table 4.8. Meeting the Daily Protein Need of an Adult at Three Cost Levels

Food	Protein, gm	Food	Protein, gm	Food	Protein, gm
1	2	3	4	5	6
		Low-Cost Menu			
Tomato juice, 1/2 c	1.0	Bean soup, ⅔ c	7.2	Meat loaf, 3 oz	21.0
Oatmeal, 2/3 c	3.3	Sandwich, peanut butter, 2T, enriched	8.0	Msh. potatoes, 3/4 c	3.0
Bread, enriched or w. w., 2 sl	4.0	or w. w. bread, 2 sl	4.0	Cabbage, 1/2 c	0.7
Nonfat milk, solids, 1 c	9.0	Carrot sticks, 1/2 c	0.6	Bread, w. w. or enriched, 2 sl	4.0
		Raw apple, 1 med	tr	Vanilla pdg., 1/2 c	4.3
		Nonfat milk, solids, 1c	9.0		
Total	17.3		28.8		33.0
		Moderate-Cost Menu			
Orange juice, frozen, 1/2 c	0.5	Mushroom soup, canned, 2/3 c	5.4	Rump pot rst., 3 oz	23.0
Egg, 1	6.0	Sandwich, cheese, 1 oz, enriched or	7.0	Msh. potatoes, 1/2 c	2.0
Bread, enriched or w. w., 2 sl	4.0	w. w. bread, 2 sl	4.0	Gr. beans, 1/2 c	1.0
Milk, 1 c	9.0	Lettuce wedge, 1/8 hd	0.5	Celery sticks, 1/2 c	0.7
		Apple betty, 1/2 c	2.0	Pan rolls, 1	3.0
		Milk, 1 c	9.0	Apricots, 2	0.5
Total	19.5		27.9		30.2

(Contd.)

1	2	3	4	5	6
High-Cost Menu					
Orange juice, fresh, 1/2 c	0.5	French onion soup, 2/3 c	0.0	Roast rib beet, 3 oz	20.0
				Baked potato, 1	3.0
Egg, 1	6.0	Sandwich, ham, 2 oz,	12.0	Asparagus, 2/3 c	2.6
Bacon, 2 sl	5.0	w. w. bread, 2 sl	4.0	Chef's salad, 2/3 c	1.0
Blueberry muffins, 1 ea	4.0	Relish plate		Cloverleaf roll, 1	3.0
		olives, pickles,		Fresh pineapple, 2/3 c	0.6
Milk, 1 c	9.0	celery, carots	0.2		
		Apple betty, 1/2 c	2.0		
		Milk, 1 c	9.0		
Total	24.5		27.2		30.2

It is fortunate that the supplementaty value of proteins makes it possible to combine cereals and legumes with dairy and meat products to provide a diet adequate in protein at comparatively low cost. The high-cost menu includes a more expensive source of meat than the moderate- and low-cost meals, that is, a rib roast as compared to a rump roast or meat loaf.

4.10. The Supplementary Value of Protein

Foods differ in the nutritive value of the protein they contain. Each food, with the exception of gelatin, contains more than one kind of protein, each with a characteristic number and concentration of amino acids. The proteins of some foods contain limited amounts of certain essential amino acids, generous amounts of others. Therefore, a combination of foods in which the amino acids contained in the proteins supplement each other is of higher nutritive quality than either alone. Early studies with experimental animals demonstrated that the proteins of milk are superior in quality to those of cereals. Nevertheless, cereal and milk fed together in the right proportions, with cereals replacing some of the milk, were as effective as milk alone. Cereals are limited in lysine; milk provides it generously.

There are possibilities of combining foods so that amino acids may supplement each other. For example, tryptophan is limited in corn and white flour, whereas foods of animal origin provide tryptophan generously. Two-thirds cup of cooked corn meal (25 gm dry) contains 0.056 gm of tryptophan, whereas a serving of pork, chicken, or beef provides approximately four times that amount. Legumes (beans and peas) are deficient in tryptophan and methionine and need to be supplemented by animal protein.

As more complete analyses are available, further possibilities of supplementation will be realized. Final conclusions on the supplementary value of certain proteins cannot be drawn, however, until it is known how will the human being is able to use the amino acids in different foods. The use of protein combinations to improve the nutritional quality of the diet holds greatest significance for persons living in parts of the world where foods of animal origin are scarce, and the diet is chiefly cereal.

Proteins and Amino Acids Worldwide

In large sections of the world and in many developing countries protein deficiency is widespread. Two-thirds of the world's population subsists almost entirely on vegetable diets such as rice, corn, wheat and cassava. In these countries the lack of animal proteins makes it necessary to develop agricultural products that will provide a mixture of plant proteins with a high nutritive value for animals and man. Much interest has been displayed in the development of an all-vegetable mixture high in protein by investigators at the Institute for Nutrition of Central America and Panama (INCAP). One of these, *Incaparina,* is being produced commercially at low cost and requires little or no readjustments in the eating habits of the native families. This formula contains 29 per cent whole ground corn, 29 per cent whole ground sorghum, 38 per cent cottonseed flour, 3 per cent Torula yeast, 1 per cent calcium carbonate, and 4500 IU of vitamin A per 100 gm. The product is sold for 3 cents for a 75 gm bag sufficient for 3 glasses (when reconstituted with water), with a protein content comparable to that of a similar amount of milk.

5

Enzymes, Digestion Absorption and Metabolism

5.1. Introduction

We all need food for our development and growth. The nutrients such as carbohydrates, fats, proteins etc., are they exist in food are not ready to be used by the body tissues in the exact form in which they are eaten. Nutrients that will ultimately be used to nourish the cells of the body are being ingested. Yet before these nutrients, present in foods, finally reach the cells, the foods themselves must be digested and the nutrients absorbed. Thus the foods that we eat must undergo some alterations in the digestive tract to fit them for absorption and assimilation. The various changes that the food undergoes in the alimentary tract are chemical and are mostly brought about mainly by the action of digestive *enzymes*.

The *digestion* of food involves the subdivision of complete molecules into simpler molecules, soluble materials (the nutrients) which can pass though digestive tract into the blood and lymph streams. After absorption the nutrients enter into the chemical processes of the body called *metabolism*.

5.2. Enzymes :

Enzymes are important group of globular proteins which act as biological catalysts in living systems.

The word *enzyme* (from the Greek "in yeast") was introduced by Kuline to refer to substances in plants or animals which had previously been called *soluble* or *unorganized* ferments to distinguish them from fermentation organisms. However, on the basis of later studies, in which more and more of activities which were previously considered to be characteristic of organism have been found to be due to enzymes, now the enzymes are commonly defined as *catalysts formed in plants and animal cells.*

Without enzymes, the living process will be too slow to sustain live. For example, without enzymes in our digestive tract it would take us same 50 years to digest a single meal. Similarly, the hydrolysis of a peptide in the laboratory requires very drastic conditions, like prolonged heating with a base but in living systems the hydrolysis of proteins occurs very rapidly in the presence of enzymes. About 3000 different hinds of enzymes have been identified so far. Some common enzymes along with their functions are listed in Table 5.1.

Table 5.1. Some Common Enzymes

Enzyme	*Reaction Catalysed*
Amy lase	Strach → Glucose
Maltase	Maltose → Glucose
Lactase	Lactose → Glucose + Galactose
Invertase	Sucrose → Glucose+Fructose
Urease	Urea → CO_2 + NH_3
Carbonic anlydrase	H_2CO_3 → CO_2 + H_2O
Pepsin	Proteins → Amino acids
Trypsin	Proteins → Amino acids
Nucleases	DNA/RNA → Nucleotides
DNA polymerases	Deoxynucleotide triphosphatco → DNA

5.3. Classification of Enzymes

Generally the enzymes are classified on the basis of the changes they help to bring about. They have been classification as:

1. The hydrolytic enzymes.
   a. Proteolytic or protein-splitting enzymes (proteases)
   b. Lipolytic or fat-splitting enzymes (lipases).
   c. Amylolytic or starch-splitting enzymes (amylases).
   d. Sugar-splitting enzymes (sucrase, maltase, lactase).
2. The coagulating enzymes, like thrombin (thrombase), which

help in the clotting of blood; and rennin, which bring about the clotting of milk.

3. The oxidizing enzymes (oxidases, dehydrogenases).

4. The reducing enzymes (reductases).

5. Those which, like the zymase of yeast, produce carbon dioxide without using free oxygen.

6. Enzymes causing the breakdown of a larger into a smaller molecule of the same composition, as in the production of lactic acid from glucose.

7. Enzymes causing chemical rearrangement without breaking down of larger into smaller molecules (mutases).

5.4. Terminology of Hydrolytic Enzymes

Duclaux suggested the each hydrolytic enzyme named in such a way that the name indicates the kind of substance on which it acts together with the suffix *ase.* Thus starch splitting enzymes are called *amylases,* fat splitting enzymes — lipases, protein splitting enzymes-proteases. The name showing the kind of change brought about or catalyzed by the enzyme is often preceded by an adjective to indicate its source: e.g., *salivary omylase* (ptyalin), *pancreatic* amylase (amylopsin). Such designation does not necessarily imply that the amylase found in the saliva either is or is not the same substance as the amylase of the pancreatic juice.

In discussion of enzymes action the substance on which the enzyme acts is called *substrate.*

Within the cell producing it, an enzyme often exists in an inactive form known as *Zymogen,* or antecedent of active enzyme. The zymogen may be stored in the cell in the form of material that gets converted into active enzyme at the time of secretion, or the secretion may be poured out with the zymogen not yet completely changed to active enzyme, or sometimes in a form that needs the presence of some other substance so as to render it active. In this case the latter substance is said to *activate* the enzyme. Activation may also mean a simple increase of activity.

5.5. Characteristics of Enzymes

Some common characteristics of enzymes are:

1. They are highly specific in their action. Each enzyme can catalyses only a specific type of reaction. For example, *maltase*

catalyses the hydrolysis of maltose. There is so other enzyme which can catalyse the hydrolysis of maltose.

2. They can speed up an uncatalysed reaction to the extent of 10 million times.

3. They are active at moderate temperature (~ 310 k) and moderate at pH 6 - 8 of the many factors which are known to influence enzyme action markedly is the hydrogen ion activity of the enzyme-substrate system. For most enzymes this must be adjusted within rather narrow limits if optimal results are to be obtained; and in some cases even to obtain any positive result. This hydrogen ion activity is commonly referred to in terms of pH, which is the symbol introduced by Sorensen to represent the negative logarithm of the hydrogen ion concentration (activity), or

$$pH = \log \frac{1}{[H^+]}.$$

As the hydrogen ion activity most favourable to the action of enzyme depends upon many interrelated factors, it should not be stated dogmatically. Remembering this, it is nevertheless of interest to note the values which have been reported as being most favourable for the action of a few of the typical enzymes. Thus, invertase (sucrase) from yeast has been reported to be most active in solutions of about pH 4.4 (Nelson), while that from the intestinal digestive juice has been found to be most active in solutions of about pH 7.0. The amylases of barley malt are most active in solutions of about pH 4.5, while that from the pancreas exerts its maximum activity in solutions of about pH 7.0 to 7.2.

With some enzymes the optimal pH is different for different substrates. Thus pepsin acting on gelatin shows a pH optimum of about 2.4, whereas when acting on casein the optimum is about pH 1.8 (Northrop, 1922). Here, and also in the case of trypsin, the changes in activity with pH seem to be related to the state of ionization of the substrate, the acid salt of the protein being most readily attacked by pepsin, the alkali salt by trypsin (Northrop, 1922). An interesting interpretation of the effect of hydrogen ion activity on enzyme activity was suggested by Michaelis for invertase (sucrase). He pointed out that the curve relating reaction velocity to pH is very similar to that relating the concentration of the unionized fraction of an amphoteric electrolyte to pH, with the optimum hydrogen ion activity for the enzyme corresponding to the isoelectric point of the ampholyte. He suggested that invertase is infact an ampholyte of which only the unionized form is catalytically active. A similar relation was found with several other enzymes, while in some cases the active form of the enzyme appeared to be ionic. Using a direct and ingenious method, Northrop (1924, 1925) showed that trypsin behaves as a univalent positive ion between pH 2 and 10, and pepsin as a univalent negative ion between pH 1 and 7. With these enzymes, the changes in activity with pH seem to be related to the state of ionization of the substrate.

4. Their action can be controlled or even inhibited by certain organic or inorganic substances.

5. Even small amounts of enzymes can be highly efficient. This is due to the fact that enzyme molecules are regenerated during their catalytic activity just like chemical catalysts.

To illustrate the point you can consider the fact that the enzymes (digestive enzymes) are capable of digesting, under favourable conditions, relatively large amounts of material. Thus pancreatic amylase when highly purified tends to lose its activity rather rapidly in solution, yet in 30 minutes at 40° C., one part of purified pancreatic amylase hydrolyzed about 20,000 parts of starch and formed about 10,000 parts of maltose (along with about an equal amount of dextrin). And in longer experiments it hydrolyzed 4,000,000 times its weight of starch with the formation of 2,800,000 times its weight of maltose before it had all become inactivated. This marked enzymic acitivity was exhibited by the preparation at a dilultion of 1 : 10,000,000 parts of water. The most delicate tests for proteins are not valid at dilutions greater than about 1 : 100,000. The purified pancreatic amylase preparation reacted like typical protein to the usual protein tests, but its own enzymic activity constituted a test for its presence which was 1000 times more delicate. Thus the failure of protein reaction in solutions enzymically achive does not show that no protein is present or that the enzyme is of other than protein nature in its chemical composition, although this negative conclusion was erroneously drawn by some investigators and repeated by many writers.

The reason that enzymes cannot hydrolyze infinite amounts of substrate is that they are themselves unstable organic substances which necessarily undergo decomposition, especially when in solution. In most cases, the purer the enzyme the more rapidly its solutions lose their activity. Another reason that an enzyme does not continue to hydrolyze substrate indefinitely is that the reaction is progressively retarded by the accumulation of the products formed.

The activity of certain enzymes may be stopped, even when all other conditions are favourable, by the accumulation of the products of the reaction; and, in certain circumstances, the action of the enzyme may be reversed so as to accelerate a change in the opposite direction to that in which it ordinarily acts.

5.6. Mechanism of Enzymatic Activity

The stepwise mechanism of enzyme catalysed reactions as proposed by Michaeli and Menten (1913) is as follows :

The reactant molecule (*substrate*) binds itself to the active site on the surface of enzyme, the active site in enzyme is so shaped that only a specific substrate can fit in it, just as a lock can be opened only with a specific key. The specific binding results in the formation of enzyme-substrate complex. Also known as *activated complex*

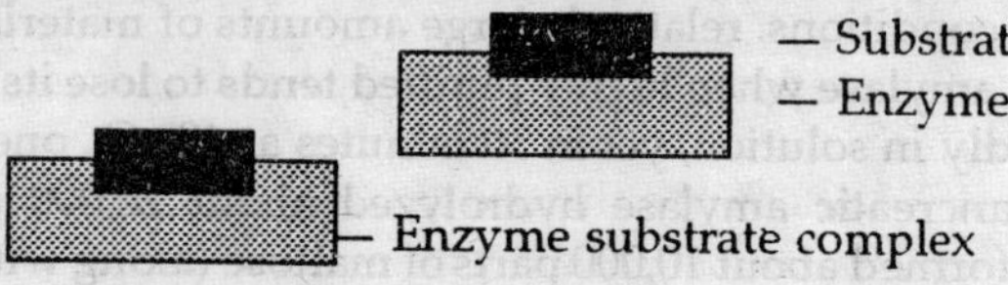

In the complex, the substrate is placed in the proper orientation to facilitate the chemical reaction and enhancing its rate. The complex finally decomposes to give products and regenerate enzymes. The general scheme can be represented as

Step I : Binding of substrate of Enzymes

$$E + S \rightarrow \{ES\}$$

Enzyme Substrate Complex

Step II : Product formation of complex

$$[ES] \rightarrow EP$$

Step III : Release of the product from the enzyme

$$EP \rightarrow E + P$$

Enzyme Product

5.7. The Chemical Nature of Some Typical Enzymes Pepsin

It was isolated in 1902 by Pekelharing. He prepared a specimen of purified pepsin and found that it contains by carbon, hydrogen, nitrogen, and sulfur in proportions within the range of variation found among ordinary proteins. It behaves like ordinary proteins in the xanthoproteic test and Millon reaction and shows the presence of the tryptophane group.

Denzani, is 1910 submitted it to hydrolyses and demonstrated that the hydrolytic products contain leucine, tyrosine, arginine, histidine and lysin. He also found evidence of other amino acids but he could not identify them because of limitations of his materials.

Northrop (1929, 1930) also established the protein nature of pepsin.

Diastase (A malt amylase)

Osborne (1895) studied its nature and observed that the enzymic activity is a property of a definite fraction of the protein material of the malt. It means that *enzyme is proteins is its chemical nature.*

In malt amylase, the enzymic activity has been found to be so inseparable from the particular protein in which it resides as to migrate with it under the influence of the electric current in either direction according to the hydrogen ion activity of the solution. Thus this enzyme shows, like other protein substances, a characteristic isoelectric point.

There is also much indirect evidence of several independent kinds supporting the view that typical enzymes are of protein nature or contain protein as a constituent, in addition to the large amount of evidence derived from investigations upon the purification of typical enzymes and study of the chemical nature of the purified preparations. And the enzyme activity has repeatedly been found to depend upon keeping the protein intact, activity being lost when the enzyme solution is subjected to treatment which coagulates, hydrolyzes, or otherwise induces chemical change in the protein matter.

We now know much about the effect of added amino acids in diminishing the rate of hydrolytic inactivation; and it is a fact that antiseptics which act chemically upon proteins are very much more destructive of the enzyme than are antiseptics of the lipoid-dissolving type. These link inactivation of the enzyme so closely and definitely with chemical change of the protein matter of the purified enzyme preparation; or, conversely, enzyme activity with intact protein.

Thus there is now abundant reason to accept the conclusion that the best-studied enzymes of the digestive tract are of protein or protein-like nature, and that food protein furnishes amino acids to serve as material for body enzymes as well as for body tissue in the more familiar sense. (To avoid even temporary misapprehension, the existence of tissue enzymes and coenzymes containing vitamin constituents may be mentioned here.

Coenzymes: Certain enzymes require non-proteinous components for their activity. There components could be metal ions like Zn^{2+}, Mg^{2+}, Mn^{2+}, Cu^{2+}, Co^{2+}, K^{+}, Na^{+} etc. or small organic molecule and are like *thiamine, niacin, riboflavin* etc. In such enzymes the protein part of the enzyme is called *apoenzyme.* Neither *coenzyme* nor *epoenzyme* can alone catalyse the reaction. The two must combine before they can act as a catalyst.

5.8. Amino Acid Derivatives as Enzymes, Hormones, or Other Nutritional Catalysts

The investigation carried out by Hopkins et al established that nutritionally essential amino acids in addition to functioning as "building stores" of the body also act as substance helpful in growth and upkeep of tissue, as precursors of hormones and also a precursors of enzymes.

To make the point clear we consider some such substance.

Glutathione

Studies conducted by Hopkins and other have shown the presence in active plant and animal tissues of an amino-acid derivative which is called glutathione. This is a tripeptide of glutamic acid, cysteine and glycine. It seems to be an important factor in the oxidation and reduction reactions of the cell, probably by virtue of the reversible change between the sulfhydryl groups (—SH) of the *cysteine* radicles in the glutathione and the disulfide groups (—S—S—) of the cystine radicals in the oxidized product. When glutathione is oxidized, two molecules containing cysteine unite to form one molecule of the oxidized product containing cystine.

The mode of linkage of the three amino acid radicles in glutathione and its corresponding structural formula, based upon its reactions and properties, were reported by Nicolet and by Kendall, Mason and McKenzie, in 1930.

Gultathione is readily soluble in water and gives an intense nitroprusside reaction which is characteristic of all active plant and animal tissues when and extract of tissue is treated with potassium nitroprusside in the presence of ammonia if the test is positive (i.e. a colour similar to that of potassium permanganate is obtained). It is probable that the reduction of nitroprusside molecule occurs. *Cysteine* (which contain sulphydryl group) gives this test but its oxidation product *cystine* does not give this test.

This test is used to follow oxidation-reduction of glutathione Hopkins pointed out that "Equilibrium in the living cell would seem to be such that the greater part of the substance (glutathione) present exists in the reduced condition; but oxidation and reduction of the constituent sulphur groups are reversible processes in the tissues, and both forms may at any moment be present." "... factors are present in the tissues which promptly reduce the oxidized product whenever its concentration is raised above an equilibrium value."

Thus, while cysteine is too unstable and reactive to exist, to an appreciable extent, as such in the tissues, it is protected in glutathione, and furnishes the reactive sulfhydryl group of this important compound. Glutathione appears to be resistant to the proteolytic enzymes of the body and to exist to an appreciable extent in all active tissues.

Thyroxine

It is an iodine-containing amino-acid derivative, obtained in the thyroid gland and then carried to the tissues of the body as a whole where it increases the rate of oxidation. It was isolated by Kendall in 1914.

It was synthesized in 1927 by Harington and Barger.

Adrenine, Adrenaline, or Epinephrine

The compound called adrenine, adrenaline, or epinephrine is the active substance formed by the adrenal (suprarenal) glands. There are differences of opinion as to its part in the oxidation processes of the body, or in the mobilization of oxidizable material. Its influences upon the rate of oxidation in the body is less marked than that of thyroxine and also more rapid and transitory. Following an injection obtadrenaline there is an almost instantaneous increase in the pasal metabolic rate of energy used which rapidly reaches a maximum and then soon drops back to normal. The entire effect, on the basal metabolic rate, of administration of epinephrine in the normal adult, is over in a few hours; whereas with thyroxine there is a well-defined delay, six to eight hours, before the basal metabolic rate is measurably increased, and the effects of a single injection upon the basal metabolic rate may still be observable for five or six weeks after the injection. Boothby has found that the extent of the increase in the rate of oxidation following the administration of epinephrine is dependent upon its concentration in the tissues.

Insulin

Insulin is concerned in the burning of glucose in the body. Insulin helps to prepare glucose for the intermediary metabolism which may lead to oxidation; not in any sense which would imply that insulin is directly an oxidizing agent.

It causes a lowering of the concentration of glucose in the blood; and this is observed both in the diabetic and in the normal body. This furnished an experimental method by which the characteristic potency of insulin concentrates was measured and progress toward the isolation of the pure substance judged. In 1926, Abel obtained it in crystalline form.

Crystalline insulin gives the typical biuret, Millon, Pauly, ninhydrin, and xanthoporteic reactions, as also specific colour reactions for several individual amino acids. So insulin, like other typical proteins, is an amino-acid derivative. The molecular, weight as indicated by the ultra-centrifuge technique is about 35,000. Jensen and Evans (1934) summarized convincing evidence that the hypoglycemic factor is identical with the crystalline protein, and not merely adsorbed or loosely bound to it. It has been pointed out that "practically the whole of this protein molecule may be accounted for in terms of a relatively few amino acids tyrosine; cystine; glutamic acid; lecuine; arginine; histidine; lysine; phenylalanine and proline. There is no special non-amino-acid constituent (prosthetic group) which would explain the unique physiological action of crystalline insulin.

The hypoglycemic effect of the hormone appears therefore to depend, if not on the entire protein molecule, at least on some certain groupings of amino acids in such molecule.

5.9. Digestion and Absorption of Food

Introduction

Began in quest of an answer to that mystery. The first notable contribution was made by Rene de Reaumur (1683-1757), a French scientist who studied changes of the food in the stomach. He performed his the next important investigations were made by Lazzaro Spallanzani (1729-1799), who studied the action of saliva on foodstuffs and verified Reaumur's observations on gastric digestion. He performed a number experiments and found that digestion takes place in human stomach. Most important were the contributions of William Beaumont (1785- 1853), a physician stationed at a military post in the forest of Northern Michigan. His observations were of the movements of the stomach during digestion and of the normal appearance of mucosa.

Food of an organism is made up of macromolecules such as proteins, fats carbohydrates etc. As they have a bigger size so the foods molecules are not diffusible and they cannot be used by body as such. They have to be broken down in diffusible particles so that they may be used by body for performing its vital functions.

A few components of diet-like salts, certain vitamins, water and other water soluble molecules are directly absorbed by the digestive tract. These however form only a small fraction of the diet.

The fragmentation of food into smaller molecules is called *digestion.*

Digestion may thus be defined as a process by which food gets altered *physically* and *chemically* into simple assimilable forms. This process can be divided into two parts (*i*) mechanical and (*ii*) chemical digestion.

The process of digestion is carried out by a number of *hydrolytic enzymes* secreted by alimentary canal and associated glands.

The Process of Digestion

The process of digestion is carried out by a number of hydrolytic enzymes secreted by alimentary canal and associated glands.

The food like the simple carbohydrates, the minerals and water can be absorbed directly because of their elementary chemical

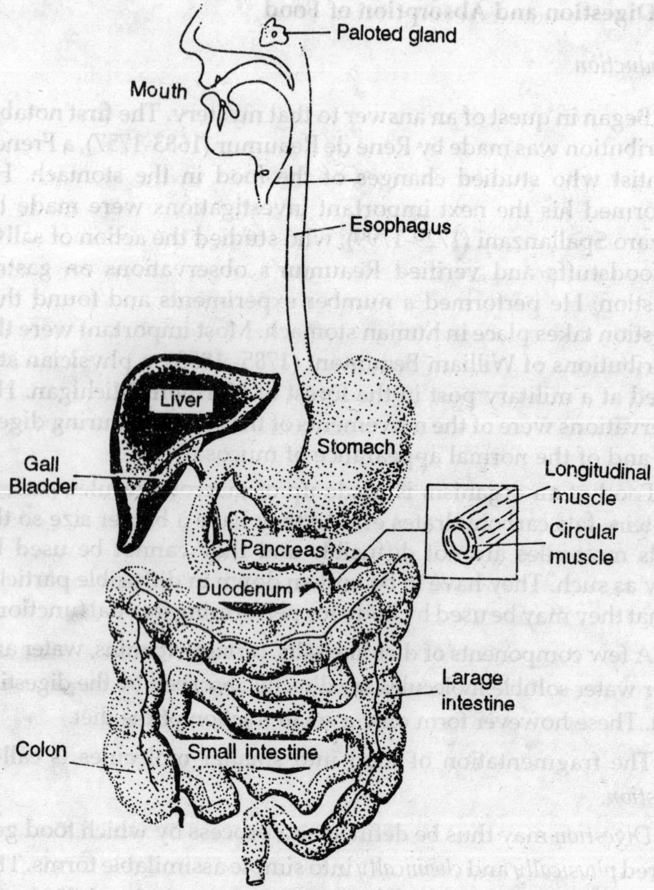

Fig. 5.1. The digestive tract.

structures. The digestion of more complex food however takes place in the gastro— intestinal tract between the mouth and the end of small intestines (Fig. 5.1). Digestion is brought about by mechanical processes and chemical action.

Food processing methods and cooking procedures actually begin the breakdown of factors in food before the food itself is ingested. Cellulose is softened and the hydrolysis of starch and collagen begin during food processing. Also cooking enhances the digestibility of some foods (egg white) and improves the flavour of others (onions). The aroma and taste of flavourful, well-prepared foods may initiate the chemical phase of digestion by stimulating the secretions of the digestive tract.

(i) Mechanical Digestion

It involves process of *liquifying* food by various digestive guices, *mastication, swallowing* and the movement of food through the tract by *peristalsis.*

Peristalsis

It is wave of muscular contraction which is preceded by a wave of relaxation that causes the contents of a hallow tube (gastrointestinal tract) to be passed on wards.

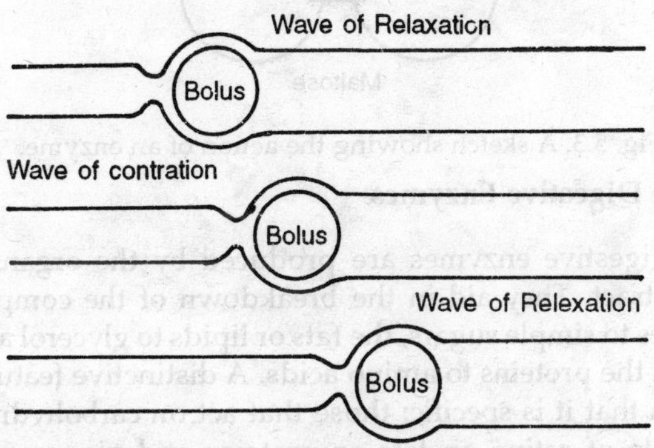

Fig. 5.2. Peristalsis.

The movements of the stomach are interfered with by nervousness and anxiety. Eating when fatigued, agitated, or worried may give rise to gastrointestinal disturbances. Hurried meals under tense conditions are not conducive to normal digestive movements.

(ii) Chemical Digestion

It is brought about by chemical substances generally *enzymes* present in various digestive juices. The process occurs when food comes in contact with such juices while passing through different levels of alimentary tract.

Some of these enzymes catalyse hydrolysis of proteins to amino acids, others of starch to monosaccharides, still others of fats to monoglycerols and fatty acids.

The following Fig 5.3, illustrates how the enzyme, maltase, aids in breaking down the disaccharide, maltose, into two molecules of the monosaccharide, glucose, without changing its own chemical structure. In addition to digestive enzymes, there are many others that are important in the body's overall function.

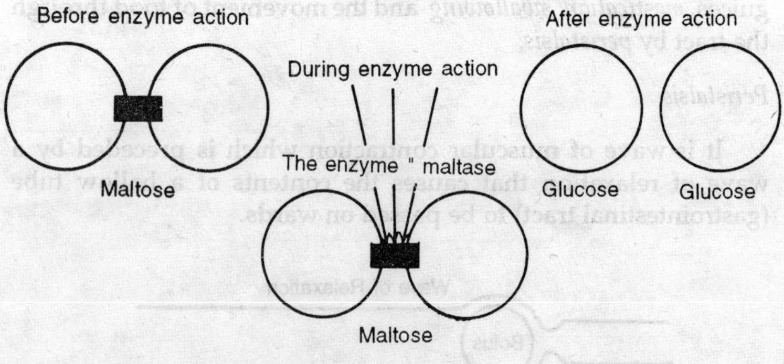

Fig. 5.3. A sketch showing the action of an enzyme.

5.10. The Digestive Enzymes

The digestive enzymes are produced by the organs of the digestive tract. They aid in the breakdown of the complex carbohydrates to simple sugars, the fats or lipids to glycerol and fatty acids, and the proteins to amino acids. A distinctive feature of an enzyme is that it is specific; those that act on carbohydrates are not capable of acting on fats or proteins and vice versa. Even though a naming system for the enzymes has been adopted, certain names which were chosen before this system was established are still in use, such as pepsin and trypsin.

The system of nomenclature adopted has already been discussed in Section 5.4.

However, the root names of the disaccharide-splitting enzymes are derived from the sugars themselves, that is *sucrase, maltase* and *lactase*. Because the steps in digestion for one nutrient may occur in different parts of the digestive tract, an adjective that describes the source of the enzymatic secretion is used before the root word to complete the enzyme name (Table 5.2). For example, the fat-splitting enzyme which acts in the small intestine is secreted by the pancreas, and is called pancreatic lipase.

Table. 5.2. The Digestive Enzymes

Source of the Enzyme Secretion	Site of Enzyme Reaction	Names of Enzymes and the Substances They Act Upon			
		Starches	Sugars	Fats	Proteins
Salivary glands	Mouth	Salivary amylase (ptyalin)			
Stomach	Stomach			Gastric lipase	Gastric protease (pepsin)
Pancreas	Small intestine	Pancr-eatic amylase		Pancreatic lipase	Pancr-eatic proteases
Wall of small intestine	Small intestine		Sucrase Maltase Lactase		intestinal proteases

Table 5.3. Summary of Chief Digestive Enzymes

	Enzymes	*Secreted by*	*Action*
Act on Carbohy-drates	Ptyalin (salivary amylase)	Salivary glands	Converts starch to maltose
	Amylopsin (pan-creatic amylase)	Pancreas	Converts starch to maltose
	Invertase (sucrase)	Intestinal mucosa	Converts sucrose to glucose and fructose
	Maltase	Intestinal mucosa	Converts maltose to glucose
	Lactase	Intestinal mucosa	Converts lactose to glucose and galactose
Act on Fats	Lipases	Gastric mucosa and pancreas	Split fats to fatty acids and glycerol

	Pepsin	Gastric mucosa	Splits proteins to proteoses and peptones
Act on Proteins	"Trypsin" (actually a group of enzymes)	Pancreas	Splits proteins to protesos, peptones, polypeptides and amino acids
	"Erepsin" (actually a group of enzymes)	Intestinal mucosa	Splits perptones to amino acids and ammonia [c]

5.11. Various Organs of Digestive System

The four important zones in which alimentary canal can be divided on the basis of physiological division of labour are—

(*i*) Ingressive zone, (*ii*) Progressive zone, (*iii*) Digestive zone, (*iv*) Egressive zone.

(*i*) In the progressive zone which includes pharynx, oscophagus and stomach the food moves forward and in this process it passes through the preliminary stages of modification.

In the digestive zone which includes small intestines the actual digestion and absorption of food occurs. It is the most part of the digestive system. In this zone the food substances passing through are diverted into the blood stream.

The *egressive zone* is represented by large intestines and extends from the termination of ileum to the anus. It brings about the expulsion of the unstable residue.

In addition to teeth, tongue and salivary glands two abdominal glands are of prime importance in the process of digestion. These are (*i*) The liver and (*ii*) the panireas.

Various parts of the digestive system are show in Fig. 5.4.

Digestion in Mouth

Food enters the digestive tract though the mouth where it is chewed, broken into small pieces, and mixed with saliva. The fluid secreted by the salivary glands contains the first of the digestive enzymes, salivary amylase (ptyalin), which hydrolyzes starch or dextrin by splitting off molecules of maltose from the long carbohydrate chain (Fig. 5.2). Furthermore the lubricating action of the saliva aids in the swallowing of the food when it passes from the mouth to the stomach by way of the *esophagus*.

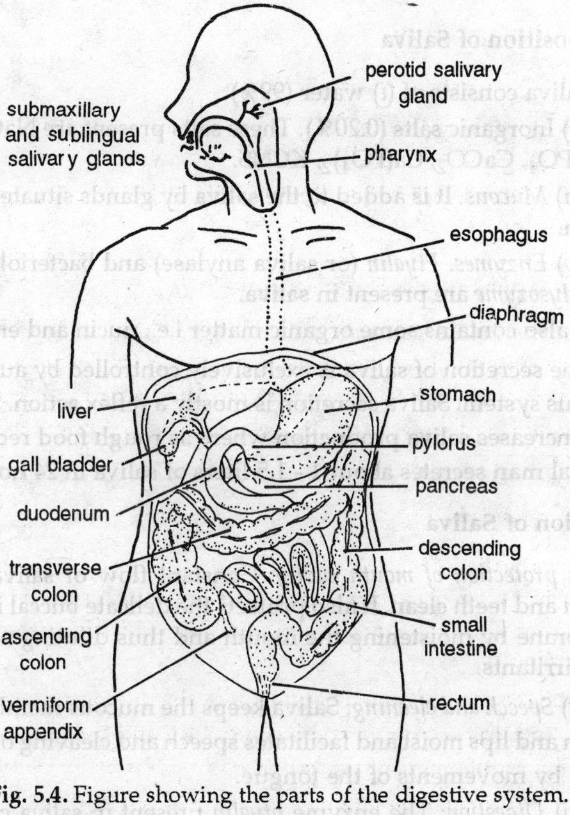

Fig. 5.4. Figure showing the parts of the digestive system.

During this process of mustication saliva is poured in the mouth by the salivary glands. The *saliva* moistens the food and forms it into a soft man or *bolus* ready for *deglutition* or swallowing. Since the saliva contains enzyme *amylase* so it hydrolyses stach into glucose and maltose.

Salivary Secretions

These pairs of salivary glands all of which are located in the mouth secrete saliva. These glands are :

(*i*) Submaxillary glands (under the angle of jaw bone)

(*ii*) Sublingual glands (under the tongue).

(*iii*) parotid glands (in front of internal openings of ear).

In addition to these some small buccal glands situated in mucosa of mouth also secret saliva.

Composition of Saliva

Saliva consists of (*i*) water (99%).

(*ii*) Inorganic salts (0.20%). These salts present are NaCl, KCl, Na_2HPO_4, $CaCO_2$, $Ca(PO_4)_2$, KCNS.

(*iii*) *Mucous*. It is added to the saliva by glands situated in the mouth.

(*iv*) *Enzymes*. *Ptyalin* (or saliva anylase) and bacteriolytic enzyme *lysozyme* are present in saliva.

It also contains some organic matter i.e., nucin and enzymes.

The secretion of saliva is exclusively controlled by automatic nervous system. Saliva secretion is mostly a reflex action. Smooth food increases saliva production where as rough food reduces it. Normal man secretes about 1 - 1.5 liters of saliva in 24 hours.

Function of Saliva

(*i*) *protection of mouth cavity*: Constant flow of saliva keeps mouth and teeth clean. It also protects the delicate buccal mucous membrane by moistening the mouth and thus diluting acid and other irritants.

(*ii*) *Speech and cleaning*: Saliva keeps the mucous membrane of mouth and lips moist and facilitates speech and cleaving of buccal cavity by movements of the tongue.

(*iii*) *Digestion*: The enzyme *ptyalin* present in saliva converts starch into sugar and thus helps into the process of digestion. The pH of saliva is 6.2-7.4.

(*iv*) *Taste*: Saliva is a good solvent and so the taste buds are stimulated by particles present in the food which are dissolved in water. It is generally observed that dry foods stimulate the sense of taste only after they thoroughly mix with saliva.

(*v*) Swallowing the very important function of saliva is its ability to moisten food and facilitate swallowing by its lubricating action.

(*vi*) *Antibacterial action*: The antibacterial enzyme *Lysozyme* present in saliva dissolves in the cell walls of many bacteria and ultimately kills them.

(*vii*) Saliva also helps in maintaining water balance of body.

(*viii*) In some animals like dog it also helps in heat regulation of body.

Deglutition or Swallowing

Deglution of swallowing is accomplished in three stages. The three stages are as under :

(*i*) The food is brought on the dorsal depressed surface of tongue by the collective action of lips, cheeks and tongue. The food bolus is pushed backwards into the pharynx by the upward movement of the tongue.

(*ii*) Food passes from pharynx into the oesophagus. Fluids pass rapidly from pharynx to oesophagus, but the solid and semisolid are pushed into oesophagus by strong constrictor muscles of pharynx.

(*iii*) The liquid passes directly from oesophagus to stomach, but the solid and semisolids are forced by peristalic actions.

The first stage is voluntary and the second and third phase is a reflex mechanism.

Digestion in the Stomach

Stomach is chiefly made up of stomach muscles. The movements of stomach are controlled by automatic nervous system. *Churning movement* brought about by three layers of muscle fibres causes mechanical break down of food, mixing of food with gastric juice and its onward movement into the duodenum. The gastric movements are of three types.

The movements of stomach besides beings under the control of automatic nervous system, are also regulated by the certain hormones. The secretion of hormones of gastro—intestinal tract depends on the chemical composition of food. The secretion of *enterogastrone* is regulated by fat content of the food. It is produced when fat rich food enters the stomach. During hunger the stomach undergoes a *peritalisis* known as *hunger contraction*. When the stomach is empty it may continue to contract. The squeezing of the empty stomach stimulates nerves in the wall and may cause hunger "pangs".

Although these contractions stimulate hunger, they have nothing to do with apetite as they quickly disappear when a small amount of food is taken.

Secretion of Gastric Juice

The stomach secrets large amounts of gastric juice which may be more than 2 litres a day. Rate of secretion is high when food is present in stomach. However, even when stomach is empty there is a continuous but slow secretion of gastric juice. There is always a small quantity of gastic juice present in the stomach even when it contains no food. This is known as *fasting juice*. Generally about 50 ml of fluid is always present in the stomach this is called *residium*.

The secretion of gastric juice is controlled by three agencies (i) the brain, (ii) the stomach and (iii) the duodenum. These three have been referred as *cephalic, gastric* and *intestinal* phases of gastric secretion.

Cephalic Phase

It is purely nervous and is meditated by vagus stimulation. This flow of juice occurs before food reaches the stomach. Sight, smell or even thought of food stimulates the cephalic centre to secrete the gastric juices.

Gastric Phase

It is both hormonal and physical and is linked with the distention of stomach rather than presence of food. Protein rich food (e.g. meat, egg, etc) stimulate the formation of hormone *gastrine* secreted by mucous of stomach. Gastrine passes directly into the circulating blood and carried to the gastric cells. It stimulates the glands in the stomach wall to produce gastric juice.

Alcohol and caffeine present in tea, coffee and cold drinks also act a stimuli for gastric release and thus acid secretion. Gastrine is also released in response to stimulation of parasympathetic fibres in the vagus nerve to the stomach.

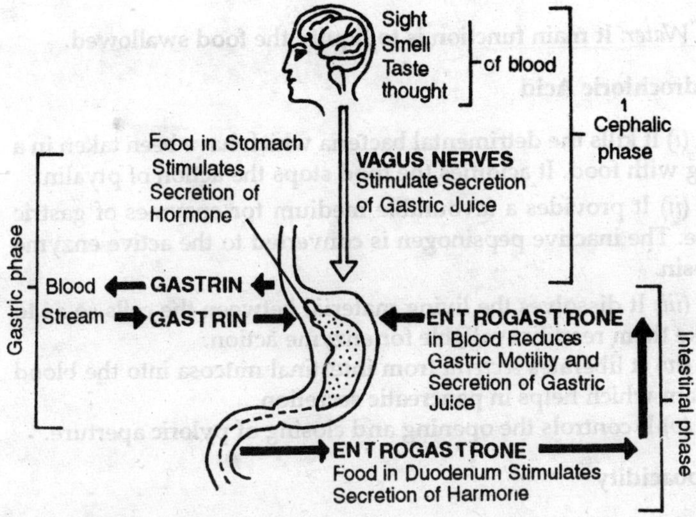

Fig. 5.5. The phases of secretion of gastric juices.

Intestinal Phase

This phase of gastric secretion is brought about when food enters the *duodenum.* It is controlled by gastrointestinal hormone. When a food rich in fats enters the duodenum, the hormone *enterogastrone* is secreted by the intestinal mucosa. This hormone enters the blood stream and then reaches the stomach where it inhibits the secretion of stomach.

Composition of Gastric Juice

The gastric juice is strongly acidic and is a mixture of substances secreted by three different types of cells. These are :

(*i*) *Parietal cells.* They secret hydrochloric acid which is approximately 0 1N and so has a pH of about 1.

(*ii*) *Mucus cells.* They produce mucus. It dilutes hydrochloric acid in the stomach and pH increases from 1 to about 1.5 or 2.

(*iii*) *Chief cells.* They produce *pepsin* and other digestive enzymes.

The mixed secretion is called gastric juice which is a clear, pale yellow fluid having a pH of about 1. It contains water (99%) hydrochloric acid (0.5%) pepsin and other digestive enzymes (e.g. rennin and gastric lipase), mucous, organic matter (0.3%), inorganic salts (3.2%), intrinsic factor.

Activities of Gastro Secretion

Water: It main function is to liquify the food swallowed.

Hydrochloric Acid

(*i*) It kills the detrimental bacteria which have been taken in a long with food. It acidifies the food stops the action of ptyalin.

(*ii*) It provides a favourable medium for enzymes of gastric juice. The inactive pepsinogen is converted to the active enzyme pepsin.

(*iii*) It dissolves the living material between the cells so as to make them readily available for enzyme action.

(*iv*) It liberates *secretin* from intestinal mucosa into the blood stream which helps in pancreatic secretion.

(*v*) It controls the opening and closing of pyloric aperture.

Hypoacidity

It refers to a condition in which the hydrochloric acid level in gastric juice is reduced. It occurs in case of gastritis, constipation, secondary anemia etc.

Hyperacidity

It refers to a condition in which the amount of hydrochloric acid secreted is more than normal. It occurs in cases of duodenal ulcer and gall bladder disease. In such a situation in pH is lowered and the rate of gastric secretion is reduced.

Enzymes

(*i*) *Pepsin*: Pepsin are a complex of four distinct enzymes Pepsin I, IIA, B, III.

Gastric pepsin is produced as the inactive zymogen, *pepsinogen*. This inactive substance is activated by HCI to *pepsin*. This transformation occurs at acidic pH. Pepsin breaks the polypeptide chain at many sites and so acts on protein to produce short peptide chains without liberating a significant quantity of amino acids.

$$\text{Pepsinogen} \xrightarrow{\text{HCl}} \text{Pepsin}$$

$$\text{Proteins} \xrightarrow{\text{Pepsin}} \text{Peptides.}$$

The pepsin transforms proteins into proteoses and peptones which are still reasonably large protein derivatives.

(ii) Rennin (Chymosin, Rennel). Rennin is inactive form and on coming in contact with HCl changes into active rennin. The optimum pH for its action is 5-6. It converts milk protein *casein* (soluble) into its insoluble form *calcium paracaseinate* (curd) in the presence of calcium.

$$\text{Rennin} + \text{Caseine} \xrightarrow{\text{Calcium}} \text{Curd.}$$

Formation of milk clot permits a longer stay for milk in stomach and also facilitates more digestion of milk proteins . This is important in the digestive process of infants because it prevents the rapid passage of milk from the stomach.

(iii) Gastric Lipase: A significant amount of weak lipolytic enzyme (gastric lipase) is present in gastric juice. It converts fats into fatty acids and glycerol. The lipolytic action of gastric juice is not important. Its activity becomes more prominent when intestinal contents are regurgitated into gastric lumen.

Mucous

It is a glycoprotein and helps in neutralising the acid in stomach. Thus it prevents high gastric acidity and injury to gastric mucosa. It acts as a lubricant.

Intrinsic Factor

Intrinsic factor (of Castle) is present in gastric juice, which is essential for the absorption of erythrocytematuring factor vitamin B_{12} (cyanocabalamin). B_{12} is absorbed with its help and carried to the liver where it gets stored. B_{12} is essential for proper development of red blood cells in bone marrow.

Regulation of Gastric Secretion

Gastric secretion is regulated by a hormone *enterogastrone* which is produced when a fat rich partially digested food reaches duodenum. This hormone when produced slows down the secretion of gastric juice and so reduces gastric motility.

Movements of Stomach

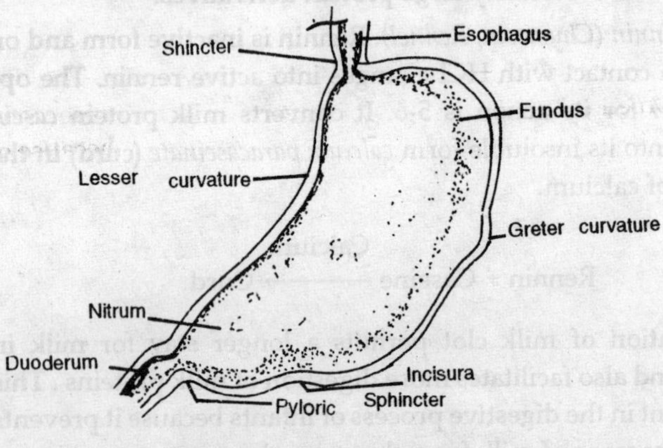

Fig. 5.6. Major features of stomach.

Major parts of stomach are shown in Fig 5.6. The stomach acts as a temporary reservoir for food and allows the digestive juices time to act an different food substances. Ordinarily meals takes five hours to leave the stomach completely. When food remains in stomach, the muscles of stomach churn the food and mix it with water and gastric juices by peristaesis waves which pass from upper part of stomach to pylorus. The peristalitic movements propel the food into the *duodenum.* The food which leaves the stomach to enter the duodenum is in semiliquid state. This partly digested food material is called *chyme.*

Digestion in Mouth

The mouth and pharynx perform two function: (*i*) mustication and (*ii*) deglutition.

When we taken the food into the mouth. The mouth is the architectural centre piece of the face. In the mouth food is chewed. In this process lower jaw is moved up wards, down wards and laterally. A combination of these movements helps in grinding the food particles. Tongue and cheeks help in the process of *mustication* (or chewing) as they help in keeping the food between teeth. The food is moved round the mouth by the tongue and the muscles of mustication.

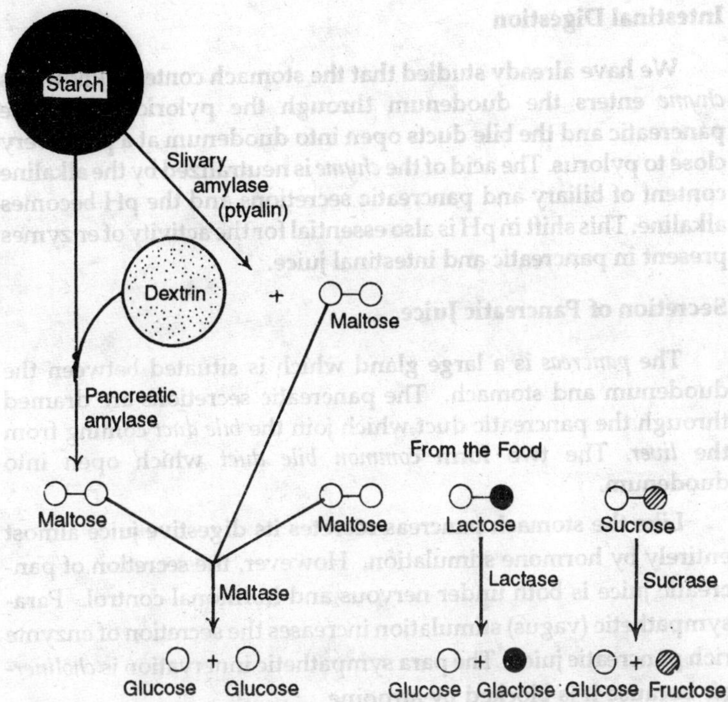

Fig. 5.7. A sketch showing starch and disaccharide digestion.

It is important to distinguish between (*a*) the elastic and relatively inactive cardiac region of the stomach, and (*b*) its muscular pyloric region—the part nearer the outlet to the small intestine.

Cannon's observations, show that the vigorous muscular movements described by Beaumont, which generally begin 20 to 30 minutes after the beginning of a meal, occur only in the middle and pyloric portion of the stomach, while the cardiac region or fundus, which serves as a reservoir for most of the food as it enters the stomach, is not actively concerned in these movements and does not rapidly mix its contents with the gastric juice.

According to Howell: "Such an arrangement of the food is more readily understood when one recalls that the stomach has never any empty space within; its cavity is only as large as its contents, so that the first portion of food eaten entirely fills it, and successive portions find the wall layer occupied and are therefore received into the interior."

Intestinal Digestion

We have already studied that the stomach contents known as *chyme* enters the duodenum through the pyloric value. The pancreatic and the bile ducts open into duodenum at a point very close to pylorus. The acid of the *chyme* is neutralized by the alkaline content of biliary and pancreatic secretions and the pH becomes alkaline. This shift in pH is also essential for the activity of enzymes present in pancreatic and intestinal juice.

Secretion of Pancreatic Juice

The *pancreas* is a large gland which is situated between the duodenum and stomach. The pancreatic secretions are dramed through the pancreatic duct which join the *bile duct* coming from the *liver.* The two form *common bile duct* which open into duodenum.

Like the stomach pancreas secretes its digestive juice almost entirely by hormone stimulation. However, the secretion of pancreatic juice is both under nervous and hormonal control. Parasympathetic (vagus) stimulation increases the secretion of enzyme rich pancreatic juice. The para sympathetic innervation is *cholinergic* because it is blocked by atropine.

When acidic chyme from the stomach reaches the intestives, the HCl in the chyme stimulates the duodenal mucous to produce a hormone known as *secretin.* The secretin has now been separated into two separate factors (*i*) Secretin and (*ii*) Pancroenzymin.

Secretin acts on pancreas which produces them pancreatic juice. This contains salt and water but no enzymes.

Pancreoenzymin works on zymogen gramules of the acinuouo cells of pancreas and stimulates the secretion of pancreatic juice which is *Lopioris* and rich in enzymes.

Composition and Functions of Pancreatic Juice

The pancreas normally produce 1-1.5 litre of juice per day. Its composition is as under

Water 99%

Inorganic matter 0.5%

Organic matter 0.5%.

Its is an alkaline fluid with pH 7—8.

The inorganic salts present are mainly those which are found in saliva or similar to them. The alkaline pH is due to the presence mainly of $NaHCO_3$.

Nature and Action of Pancreatic Enzymes

It has the following hydrolytic enzymes.

(*i*) *Trypsin*: It is secreted as *tripsinogen*: (inactive form) which gets converted into active form *trypsin* on contact with intestinal mucous (*enterokinase*). It is made up of 233 amino acid molecules and has a mol. wt. of 34,000. Its optimum activity is in pH 8-9. In alkaline medium it hydrolysis proteins yielding various polypeptides and a few amino acids. The activity of *trypsin* can be inhibited by egg white, human and vovine *colostrum*.

(*ii*) *Chymotrypsin*: It is secreted in the inactive form *chynrotryprinogen* which becomes active in alkaline medium (pH=7-9) in the presence of *trypsin*. *Chymotrypsin* has more coagulating power for milk than trypsin. It attacks peptide links with adjacent aromatic amino-acids. It is inhibited by organic phosphates like isoprophylfluoro phosphate and benzoyal derivative of some amino-acids.

Amylases or Amylopsin

This is the carbohydrate hydrolysing enzyme. The starch splitting action of pancreatic juice is due to pancreatic *alpha-amylase*. Its optimum activity pH range is 6.2 -7.2. For *amylase*, chloride and phosphate act as coenzymes. Its action is similar to salivary amylase.

$$\text{Amylase} + \text{starch, Glycogen} \rightarrow \text{Maltose.}$$

The presence of Lactase, Sucrase and Maltase has also been reported

$$\text{Lactose} \xrightarrow{\text{Lactase}} \text{Glucose} + \text{Galactose}$$

$$\text{Sucrose} \xrightarrow{\text{Sucrase}} \text{Glucose} + \text{Fructose}$$

$$\text{Maltose} \xrightarrow{\text{Maltose}} \text{Glucose.}$$

Lipase or Steapsin

It is the fat splitting enzyme of pancreatic juice and is secreted in the active form. Fats are hydrolysed by pancreatic lipase to fatty acids and glycerol.

Lipase + Emulsified Fats → Fatty acids and Glycerol.

Its action is highly promoted by bile salts, soaps, calcium salts and some peptides. It is inhibited by quinine and some other alkaloids. The optimum in activity is in pH 7-8.

Pancreatic juice also contains *phospholipase* called *lecithinase* and *cholesterol-esterase.*

Carboxypeptidases

These are found in pancreatic juice in the inactive form *procarboxypeptidase.* They get converted into the active form in the presence of *trypsin* and *enterokinase.* They act best on peptides containing tyrosine, phenylanalin or tryptophan.

Pancreopeptidase E or Elastase

This enzyme hydrolyses elastin and can also drydrolyse many other proteins.

Nucleolytic Enzymes

Pancreatic juice contains two enzymes which can hydrolyse RNA and DNA. These are *Ribonuclease* or RNAse which dissociates RNA into its components and simple nucleotides and *Deoxyribonuclease* or *dorase* or *DNAse* which dissociates DNA into its components or simple nucleotides.

Intestinal Juices

The intestinal juice is secreted by two distinct type of glands found in small intestines. (*i*) the duodenal glands and (*ii*) the intestinal glands or crypts of Lieberkuhn.

The crypts of Liberkuhn contain a number of different types of cells secreting large number of enzymes. These enzymes are collectively called *success entericus.* It is a clear yellow fluid secreted in amount of about 2-3 litre per day. It has a pH of about 7.8. This is the digestive juice which completes the digestion of carbohydrates, proteins and fats.

Simulation of Intestinal Secretion

When *chyme* enters the small intestines it stimulates the mucous membrane to secrete the hormone *enterocrinin*. This induces the flow of intestinal juice from intestinal glands.

Composition and Functions of Intestinal Juice

Intestinal juice contains about 98.5% water, 1.5% solid matters, mucus and enzymes. Mineral salts generally present in it are Cl^- HCO_3^-, PO_4^{3-} of Na^+, K^+, Ca^{2+} and Mg^{2+}.

Enzymatic Activities

The important enzymes and their functions are given below :

Enzyme	*Function*
(*i*) *Enterokenase*	Converts inactive *Trysinogen* to active trypsin.
(*ii*) *Erepsin*	Converts tri- and di-peptides to mono-peptides (amino acids).
(*iii*) *Invertase*, (*Sucrase*)	Converts sucrose into glucose and fructose.
(*iv*) *Maltase*	Converts Maltose into fructose.
(*v*) *Lactase*	Converts Lactose into Glucose and Galactose.
(*vi*) *Lipase*	Converts emulsified fats into fatty acids and glycerol.
(*vii*) *Phospholipase*	Converts phospholipids to Glycerol, fatty acids and phosphoric acid.
(*viii*) *Phosphatase*	Converts organic phosphate to free phosphate.
(*ix*) *Polynucleotidase*	Converts nuclear acids to nucleotides.
(*x*) *Nucleosidases*	Converts *purine* or *pyramidine* nucleosides to purine or pyramidine bases, pentose phosphate.

The Bile

Liver continuously secrets a juice known as *bile*. *Bile* is collected by a number of hepatic ducts which join together to form the *common heptic duct*. This immediately joins the duct from the gall bladder (cystic duct) and continues towards the intestine as the *bile duct*.

Bile is an alkaline, viscous, yellow green bitter fluid (pH=8.6). Human bile is yellowing green, in carnivora its colour is golden yellow, in herbivora its colour is green.

Some quantity of *bile* is stored in the gall bladder. On digestion gall bladder contracts and supplies *bile* rapidly to small intestines.

Gall bladder bile contains about 86.0% water and 14.0% salts (8% of bile salts are sodium salts of glycocholic acid and taurocholic acid, 2% bile pigments and mucin, 3% cholesterol and other lipids and 1% inorganic salt).

Secretions of Bile

The release of bile is controlled by a hormone *cholecyst okini*. This hormone is produced by mucosa of upper intestines, when fats and acid enter the intestines. The hormone enters the blood stream and causes.

Role of Bacteria in Intestines

The intestine of a new born child is found to be sterile and excretes a semifluid mass called *meconium*. Only after a few days the intestine is invaded and colonised by ingested bacteria. Small intestine has a substanial flora mostly of *streptococci, lactobacilli* and *fungi*. Another type of organism are found in lower small intestine which are similar to those found in colon (e.g., amaerobes, etc.).

Food stays in colon for about 3 hours and the microorganisms carry out *fermentation* and *putrefaction*. In these processes polysacharides are changed into similar substances (fermentation) and proteins are changed into similar substances (putrefaction).

The microorganisms can also bring about the utillization of ammonia and urea for the synthesis of proteins. In human beings intestinal bacteria can synthesize vitamin A, B-complex, D and K.

Absorption from the Gastro Intestinal Tract

Absorption is the third phase of physiological processes occurring in alimentary tract. The first two being Ingestion and digestion.

Absorption from the Mouth

Only a few drugs may be absorbed into the blood through the mucous membrane in the mouth. e.g. *isoprenaline, glyceryl trinitrate*. These drugs are absorbed only when allowed to dissolve under the tongue.

Absorption from the Stomach

In stomach limited absorption can take place. The only substances likely to be absorbed in stomach are water, glucose and alcohol. They get absorbed through the walls of the stomach into the venous circulation.

Some iron absorption occurs in small intestines but it is dissolved out of food most effectively in the stomach in presence of HCl.

Absorption from small Intestines

Small intestines is the main absorption organ and about 90% of the ingested food get absorbed here. The large surface area of intestines provides more opportunities of absorption the simultaneous contraction and relaxation of sphincter of oddi.

Although the release of bile is generally controlled by cholecyst okinin (CCK), the vagus nerve also exercises a control on its opening. Stimulation of vagus nerve causes *spasin* in the sphincter of oddi. If the vagus nerve is cut gall bladder empties slowly.

Functions of Components of Bili

Mineral salts present in bile neutralize the acid chyme from the stomach.

Bile salts brings about emulsification of fats in the duodenum. In this process fat globules break down into a suspension of very fine droplets I *μm* in diameter. This provides larger surface area for enzymes lipase to act upon and quickens the process of digestion. Bile salts also help to bring down the surface tension of water. Bile is essential for the adsorption of fat soluble vitamins (i.e. vitamin A, D, E and K). Bile salts also participate in *'enter-hepatic circulation'* of bile salts.

Mucous acts as a lubricant and as a buffer cholesterol and *Lecithin* are chiefly excertory products. Bile is also an important vehicle of excretion.

The absorbed material in intestines is transported either by the veins of the *hepatic portal system* into the liver or by *lymphatic vessals* to the blood.

Absorption of Carbohydrates

Carbohydrates are broken down and absorbed in the form of monosaccharides. The digested carbohydrates are absorbed through the intestinal villi. The small intestine is the main absorptive organ. About 90% of ingested food stuff is absorbed while it passes through the small intestine.

There are two mechanisms of absorption in intestines. These are (*i*) *diffusion* and (*ii*) *active absorption*. There are two general path ways for the transport of material absorbed by the intestines. These are: (*i*) *the veins of the hepatic portal system, (ii) the lymphatic vessels of the intestinal area.*

The rate of absorption of different sugars (monosaccharides) has been found to be in the following order galactose > glucose > fructose > mannose > xylose > arbinose etc.

Pentoses have smaller molecules and so can diffuse more rapidly as compared to hexoses.

Monosaccharides are absorbed by active transport. The absorption depends upon presence of Na^+ ions.

Fructose is transported by simple diffusion in response to a concentration gradient by absorptive cells of the villi.

Glucose and lactose are actively transported. It is postulated, that in the active absorption of glucose, a mobile carrier binds both glucose and Na^+ ions separate sites and transports them both through the plasma membrane of the intestinal cell. It releases sugar inside the cell. Carrier needs energy. Na^+ effects the supply of energy from ATP probably by activating AT Pase are in the cell membrane. The carrier compound is first phosphorelated with ATP and the sugar combines with phosphoric acid to form hexose phosphate. Before entering the blood hexose phosphate gets hydrolysed and so we find hexose and not hexose phosphate in blood.

Absorption of Aminoacids and Proteins

At the end of protein digestion most of the proteins get converted into amino acids by the action of *proteases* and a small part is left in the form of small polypeptides.

Amino acids are absorbed into the intestinal cappillaries and these enter the portal veins from where it is carried to the circular-tory system. Different carrier system exist for transporting different classes of amino acids. Some of these require Na^+ just as in case of carbohydrates.

The amino acids are absorbed at different rates which depend on mol. wt. of the amino acid. Glycine is absorbed more rapidly, alaline, cystine, glutamic acid, valine etc. follow it in the above order.

Generally L-amino acids are absorbed more rapidly than the corresponding D-isomer.

Very little quantity of proteins is also absorbed by *pinacytosis*. This does not have any nutritional value. In certain cases, some of the unchanged proteins can act as *antigens* for forming *antibodies*. When sufficient quantities of antibodies are producer further absorption of protein produces a reaction in the form of *ashes* or *asthmatic* conditions. An individual is then said to be *allergic* to a particular protein.

Absorption of Fats

Fats get hydrolysed to yield a mixture of glycerol, diglycerides, monoglycerides, fatty acids by the action of *pancreatic lipases* during digestion. These products of fat digestion enter the mucosal cells of small intestines.

The absorption of fatty acids depend upon their mol.wt. (*i*) the short chain and water soluble long chain fatty acids are directly absorbed through the absorptive cells of intestines into portal blood system, (*ii*) the unbroken fatty acids and glycerides, which are in the form of *miscelles* are absorbed through *crypts* between the microvilli of intestinal absorptive cells. From the crypts the fats are transferred into the cytoplasm through *pinocytosis*.

The fatty acids can also be absorbed in combination with the steroids by forming more soluble esters. As soon as absorption occurs, this complex breaks down, the fatty acids liberated from complex, and the bila salt is finally carried to the river, where it is re-secreted in the bile. Experimentally it has been found that if fats are fed to an animal whose bile duct has been tied off, about 80 per cent of fatty acids are found in the faeces.

The absorbed or resynthesized long chain fatty acids enter the lymphatic system as triglycerides particularly in the form of *chylomicrons*. The chylomicrons are about one micron in diameter and are made up of 2% protein, 7% phospholipid, 9% cholesterol, and 82% triglycerides. The particles of emulsified fat having dimensions 0.1 to 0.5% are known as the micelles that can be easily absorbed as such without undergoing hydrolysis. In some cases because of biliary obstruction and liver dysfunction, there is a loss of the absorbed fats through urine. The urine becomes milky and the condition is called *chyluria*. Sometimes fats may pass into the peural fluid causing *chylothorax*. In this case also pleural fluid becomes milky.

In short the digestion of fat takes place only to make the complex molecule diffusible through the intestinal villi, because the digested products are reconverted again into the natural fats as were present in the food.

Absorption of Vitamins

Water-soluble Vitamin such as the members of B Complex (except B_{12}) and vitamin C readily diffuse across the walls of the intestine into the blood. To move vitamin B_{12} across the wall of the ileum, a special system is needed. In the stomach, the vitamin combines with a special protein secreted by the gastric glands, called the *intrinsic factor*. During the absorption process in the ileum, Vitamin B_{12} is released from the intrinsic factor and enters the blood.

The *fat-soluble vitamins*, A, D, E and K are dissolved in micells that enter the mucosal cells of the intestine by simple diffusion. The absorption of these fat-soluble vitamins is markedly decreased in the absence of bile.

Absorption of Nucleic Acids

Nucleic acids are first hydrolyzed in the gut into nucleosides of RNA and DNA in the presence of ribonuclease and deoxyri bonuclease respectively. Thus nucleoside is the diffusable form of nucleic acid.

Absorption of Water and Electrolytes

In human being about 15-20 litres of water can be absorbed in ileum in one day. The process of movement of water in the intestine is known as the *gastro intestinal circulation*.

The mucosa of large intestine is the main organ for the sodium absorption. Chloride is absorbed along with the sodium ions. Iron is absorbed in the duodenum while calcium a long the entire length of the intestine. The absorption of calcium is 50 times slower as compared to that of the sodium. Bicarbonate is absorbed by different areas of the intestine.

Functions of the Large Intestine

When the contents of small intestines enter the large intestines they are mostly in semiliquid form and are made up of undigested food, and remains of digestive juices. Much of the water of the intestinal contents is absorbed here. The contents of the large intestines are called *faeces.*

The large intestines secretes mucin. Mucin help to liberate faeces and in this way facilitates its passage through rectum and anus.

The absorption of water from the food residue as it passes through the large intestines helps to maintain the balance of body water. Some minerals and salt may also get slowly absorbed in large intestines.

Large intestines also help in excretion of excess of calcium, iron and drugs of heavy metal type like bisminth, etc.

Bacterial decomposition of cellulose also occurs in large intestines. The faecai matter remains stored in large intestines for about 35 hours during which it is acted upon by a number of bacteria which impart faeces their characteristic foul smell.

Deflecation

Mass peristaltic movement pushes faecal matter into the rectum. The resulting distension of the rectal wall stimulates pressure sensitive receptors initiating a reflex which is *gastrocolic reflex* or *defecation*, which is emptying of the rectum.

The act of defecation, while reflex in infants, in the adult is under the control of the will. Defecation is controlled by the inner and outer sphincter muscles which encircle the anus. The inner sphincter is involuntary but the outer sphincter is voluntary.

The following actions occur during defection :

1. The sphincter muscle of the anus relaxes.

2. The muscular walls of the rectum contract.
3. The muscles of the floor of the pelvis contract.
4. The pressure within the abdomen is raised.

The frequency of defecations is variable from person to person.

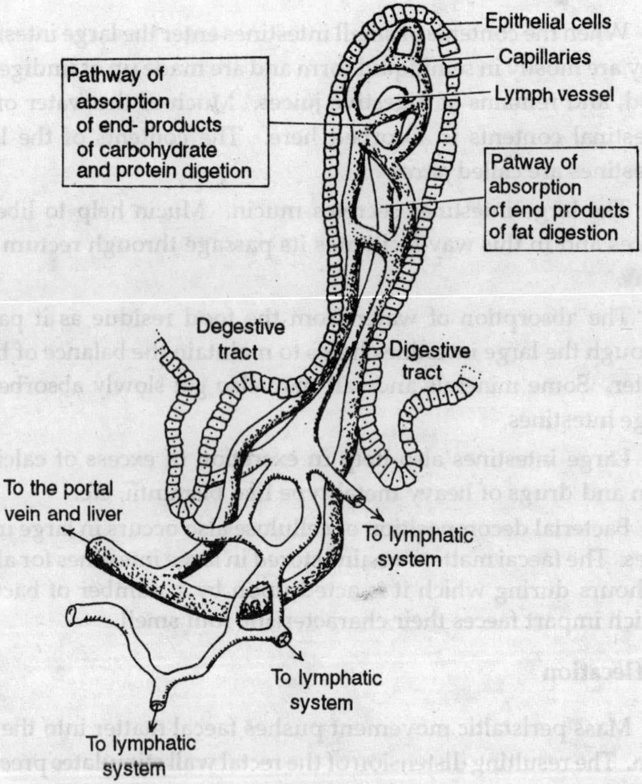

Fig. 5.8. A sketch of a villus, the absorptive organic of the small intestine.

5.12. Coefficients of Digestibility of Food

The fecal matter passed per day varies considerably in health, but on an ordinary mixed diet of reasonably digestible food materials is usually between 100 and 200 grams of moist substance containing 25 to 50 grams of solids. The feces contain any undigestible substances swallowed with the food and any undigsted residues of true food material; but ordinarily they appear to be largely composed of residues of the digestive juices, together with certain substances which have been formed in metabolism and excreted by way of the intestine, and bacteria, living and dead.

The experiments performed by Prausnitz showed that although the solids of the meat were about ten times as rich in nitrogen as the solids of the rice the two diets yielded feces whose solids were of nearly the same composition. Thus the nitrogen compounds feces represent material either lost or expended in the work of digestion so the nitrogen of the feces be deducted from that of the food in estimating the amount available for actual tissue metabolism. This however in by no means equally true of the mineral elements, some of which, after being metabolized in the body, are eliminated mainly by way of the intestine rather than through the kidneys.

On a liberal diet consisting entirely of non-nitrogenous food, the amount of nitrogen in the feces was 0.5 to 0.9 gram per day, which is more than is sometimes found in feces from food furnishing enough protein to meet all the needs of the body. Thus the expenditure of nitrogenous material in the digestion of fats and carbohydrates may be larger than in the digestion of protein food.

The feces always contain ether-soluble substances as well as protein. Fasting men have eliminated 0.6 to 1.3 grams per day of total lipids, a large part of which was sterols.

When the diet is very poor in fat and other lipids, the feces may contain as much as was contained in the food. As the fat content of the food rises, the actual amounts in the feces increase, but the relative amounts decrease so that up to a certain point the apparent percentage utilization of the fat becomes higher. The limit to the amount of fat which can be thus well digested varies with the individual and with the form in which the fat is given. Quantities up to 200 grams per day have been absorbed to within 2 to 3 per cent when given in the form of milk, cheese, or butter.

In addition to protein and the fat the feces always contain various other forms of organic matter which in the routine proximate analyses usually made in connection with feeding experiments are collectively reported as "carbohydrates determined by difference."

With these facts in mind one may make use of the coefficients of digestibility without being misled by them. These coefficients show the relation between the constituents of the food consumed and the corresponding constituents of the feces. Thus if the feces from a given diet contain 5 per cent as much protein as was contained in the food, this proportion is assumed to have been lost or expended in digestion, and the coefficient of digestibility of the protein of the diet is started to be 95 per cent. While, as just shown this assumption is not entirely correct, yet it is approximately true of the organic nutrients that the difference between the amounts in the food and in the feces represents what is available to the tissues of the body, and thus these coefficients serve a useful purpose in the computation of the nutritive values of foods.

From the results of hundreds of digestion experiments Atwater computed the average coefficients of digestibility of the organic nutrients of the main group of food materials, when used by man as part of a mixed diet, to be as shown in Table 5.4.

Table 5.4. Average Coefficients of Digestibility of Foods When Used in Mixed Diet (Atwater)

	Protein Per cent	*Fat Per cent*	*Carbohydrate Per cent*
Animal foods	97	95	98
Cereals and breadstuffs	85	90	98
Dried legumes	78	90	97
Vegetables	83	90	95
Fruits	85	90	90
Total food of average mixed diet	92	95	98

In some cases, these figures are higher than have been reported for similar foods by other observers, the differences being due mainly to the fact (not formerly recognized) that a food may be more perfectly utilized when fed as a part of a simple mixed diet than when fed alone. Milk is an example of such a food, and has, when consumed as part of a mixed diet, a much higher coefficient of digestibility than is often assigned to it on the basis of earlier experiments.

It will be seen that the coefficients differ less for the different types of food than might be expected from popular impressions of "digestibility" and "indigestibility". It is also noteworthy that the coefficients of digestibility are less influenced by the conditions under which the food is eaten and vary less with individuals than is generally supposed. In explanation of this it may be said that general impressions of digestibility relate mainly to ease or comfort of digestion, which often bears little relation to the extent to which the food is ultimately digested in its passage through the entire digestive tract.

5.13. Metabolism

Metabolism may be described as all the chemical changes that nutrients undergo from the time they are absorbed until they become a part of the body or are excreted from the body. The two general phases of metabolism are referred to as *anabolism* and *catabolism*. The anabolism phase involves all the chemical reactions that the nutrients undergo for the construction or building up of body materials such as blood, enzymes, various tissues, hormones, glycogen and others. The catabolism phase involves the reactions in which various compounds of the tissues are broken down, such as carbohydrates into carbon dioxide and water, releasing energy. In the cell both processes go on simultaneously. *Energy metabolism* is the general term that has come to be used to describe all the changes, both chemical and physical, that the energy nutrients undergo in the release of energy for the body's use.

Enzymes of Metabolism as Distinguished from Digestion

Just as the organic reactions of our digestive processes are largely catalyzed, so are those of our metabolic processes. Thus, more or less parallel with the digestive enzymes are the tissue respiratory enzymes. And a number of body substances which catalyze other types of reaction may also properly be called enzymes and (or) given names ending in *ase* if one wishes. There seems (1951) to be a trend in this direction, and to explain the organic reactions of the intermediary metabolism in enzymatic terms.

Carbohydrate Metabolism

After the end products of carbohydrate digestion (the monosaccharides) reach the liver, they are used for energy or stored, depending on the body's immediate need. There is evidence that monosaccharides, except glucose, are changed to glucose in the liver cells. These glucose molecules are sent to all parts of the body via the blood stream and pass from it into the tissues and cells by way of the fluids that surround the cells. The carbohydrate is oxidized in the cell to supply energy needed for the body processes.

The Formation of Glycogen

The formation of glycogen from glucose in either the liver or muscle cells involves a series of enzymatic reactions. In one of these chemical steps, the catalytic agents involved are ions of

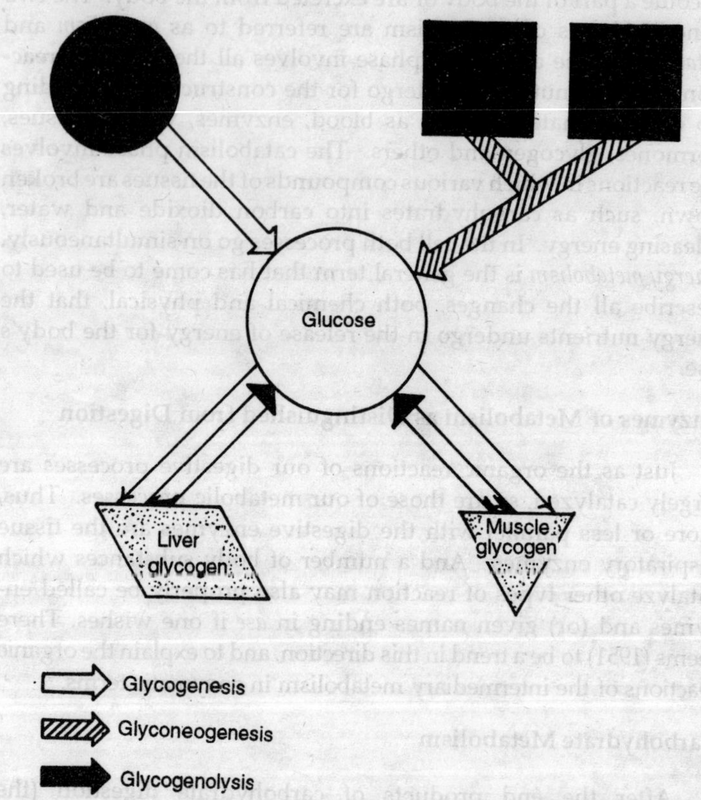

Fig. 5.9. A sketch depicting the formation of glucose and glycogen.

magnesium. The glycogen formed, often referred to as animal starch, is stored both in the liver and in the muscle. However, only limited amounts of this complex carbohydrate can be stored as compared to the body's storage capacity for fat. It has been estimated that the liver can store up to 10% of its weight in glycogen or about 100 gm, and the storage capacity of the muscle is only about 2% of its weight.

Insulin plays an essential role in carbohydrate metabolism. This hormone, which is secreted by the Islets of Langerhans of the pancreas, aids not only in the oxidation of glucose in the body, but also accelerates the conversion of blood glucose to glycogen.

The Breakdown of Liver and Muscle Glycogen

When extra energy is needed by the body, the liver glycogen is mobilized and changed to glucose by a process called glycogenolysis (Fig. 5.9). This reaction occurs only in the liver cells. *Epinephrine,* commonly referred to as *adrenalin,* is the hormone produced by the adrenal glands which stimulates the breakdown of liver glycogen. After the glucose has been formed, it leaves the liver and passes to the tissues for immediate use.

The breakdown of muscle glycogen also is accelerated by adrenalin. However, the end product of this conversion is not glucose but a closely related compound, glucose-I-phosphate.

Glucose Formation from Noncarbohydrate Sources

Although most of the glucose in the body comes from dietary carbohydrates, it may be formed in the liver from noncarbohydrate molecules by a process called glyconeogenesis (Fig. 5.8). The three sources of noncarbohydrate molecules, which may be precursors of liver glycogen and finally blood glucose, are the glycerol part of fat molecules, *deaminized amino acids,* and other compounds along the glycolytic pathway (e.g., lactic acid). A deaminized amino acid is one in which the amino group NH_2 has been removed.

Oxidation of Carbohydrate for Energy

The steps in the oxidation of carbohydrate for energy are pictured in Fig. 5.9. The first stage in the oxidation process involves the breakdown of glycogen or glucose to pyruvate (pyruvic acid) and lactate (lactic acid). This conversion is not a simple chemical change but occurs in many complex enzymatic reactions. In addition to this a derivative of the glycerol part of the fat molecule enters the oxidation on cycle along the glycolytic pathway.

The second stage in the oxidation process involves the breakdown of pyruvate to carbon dioxide and water with the release of energy. Energy is released when one molecule pyruvate goes through the complete cycle of the chemical changes known as the Kreb's Cycle. Oxygen is required in these reactions.

Even though the exact mechanism found in the oxidation process is complicated and involved, the sketch gives an idea of the series of known reactions that take place in this complex process.

Conversion of Carbohydrates to Fats and Amino Acids

When carbohydrates are ingested in quantities greater than the energy needs of the body, the excess amount is converted to fat and stored in the tissues. This fact has been demonstrated by controlled experiments with both animals and men. From the sketch (Fig. 5.10) it can be seen how a fat may be formed from a carbohydrate. The glycolytic pathway from carbohydrate to glycerol and from the "acetyl CoA" (a coenzyme concerned with enzymatic processes involving two-carbon compounds) to fatty acid are both two-way reactions. Derivatives of either glycogen or glucose may be diverted from the main pathway and travel along these side reactions to glycerol and fatty acids. These two substances then combine to form a fat which is stored in the body tissue.

Besides being converted to fat, extra carbohydrate may also assist in the formation of amino acids. It can be seen how it is possible for this to occur from the sketch of the chemical system. For example, pyruvate may be oxidized to release energy, reconverted to carbohydrate, used for the synthesis of fat, or synthesized into an amino acid. It is here that the synthesis of the amino acid alanine occurs. Two other amino acid derivatives, glutamate (glutamic acid) and aspartate (aspartic acid), are synthesized also from pyruvate. Then glutamate gives rise to proline, hydroxyproline, arginine and histidine. It is of interest that the chemical reactions involving four nonessential amino acids (serine, cysteine, glycine and tyrosine) and the six essential amino acids (threonine, valine, methionine, leucine, isoleucine, and phenylalanine) constitute only one-way reactions to either pyruvate or acetyl-CoA.

Fat Metabolism

After the end products of fat digestion are absorbed through the walls of the intestinal tract, they pass into the lymph vessels on their way to the cells and tissues. Later they enter the blood stream, but before doing so some of the recombined fat molecules unite with molecules of phosphoric acid to form phosphor, which aid in the transport of fatty acids in the body. The recombined fats, the phospholipids, the glycerides, the glycerol molecules, and the fatty acids go to all the body tissues, where they are either oxidized for energy or stored as adipose or fatty tissue.

Oxidation of Fats: The components of a fat molecule, the glycerol fraction, and the fraction of fatty acids, are oxidized separately to provide energy for the body processes. Before oxidation can begin, therefore, any fat or glyceride must first be hydrolyzed to glycerol and fatty acids.

The glycerol part of the fat molecule is first changed to a new compound before it enters the glycolytic pathway midway between the point marked "carbohydrate" and that marked "pyruvate" in Fig. 5.10. From here on the oxidation of glycerol is the same as the oxidation of carbohydrate.

The fatty acids, however, undergo several changes before they reach the acetyl-CoA reaction. From this point they travel the same route along the Kreb's Cycle as do the carbohydrates and the glycerol fraction of the fat in order to release carbon dioxide, water, and energy.

Fat Formation from Carbohydrates and Amino Acids: Both carbohydrates and amino acids may be used as sources of fat in the body. The formation of body fat from carbohydrates has already been mentioned. The conversion of protein to body fat, however, involves the amino acids along the metabolic pathway. As seen in Fig. 5.10, the amino acids are first deaminized and then proceed to acetyl-CoA. From this point they proceed to fatty acids as well as to pyruvate and then to the point where the reaction leads off to glycerol. The glycerol and fatty acid molecules then combine to form a glyceride.

The amino acids, the end products of protein digestion, are readily absorbed into the blood stream from the intestinal mucosa,

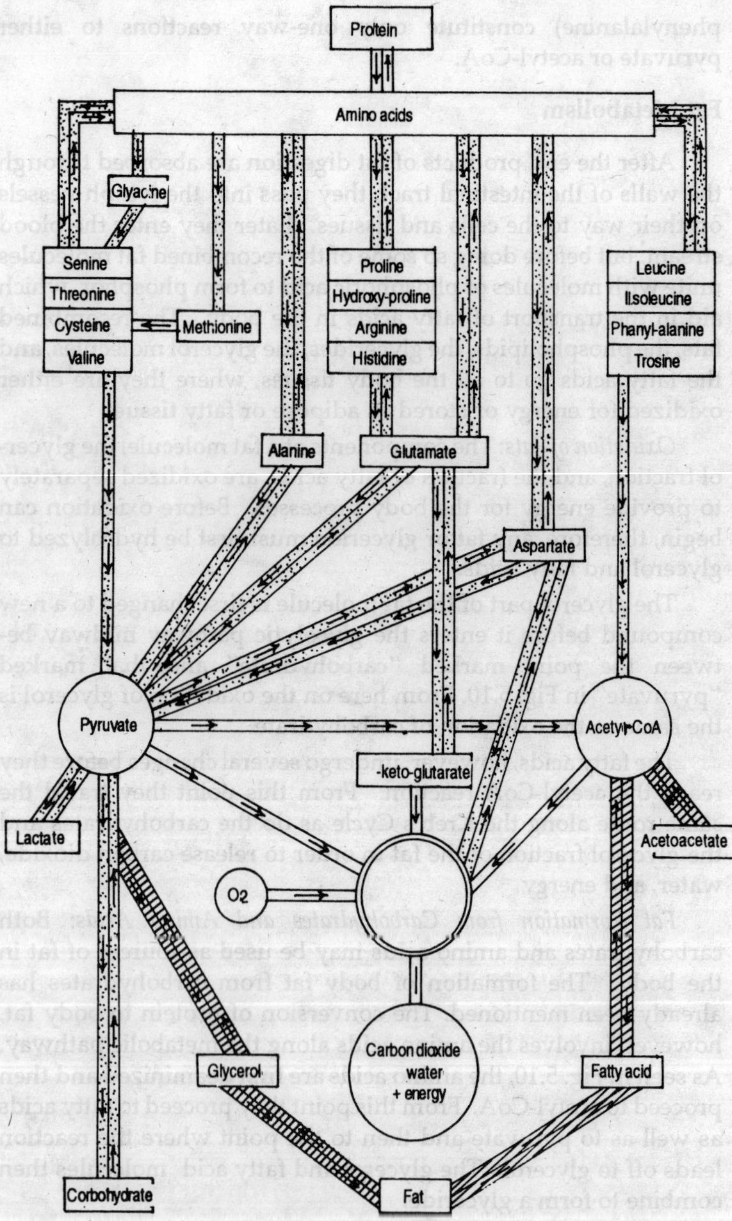

Fig. 5.10. A sketch depicting the chemical system which represents the pathway of oxidation for carbohydrates, fats, and proteins in the body.

pass to the liver, and from there are carried to all the cells of the body. There are three ways in which the amino acids are used by the body. First, some are synthesized to proteins and are used by the body to build new cells and to replace worn -out ones and to form body regulators, that is, hormones, enzymes, antibodies. Second, some of the amino acids may exchange amino groups with other amino acids or even contribute amino groups to non-protein materials to form new amino acids. Finally, amino acids may undergo oxidation for energy production.

Formation of Body Protein: A discussion of factors related to protein formation in the body.

Oxidation of Amino Acids: Before amino acids enter the metabolic pathway to be oxidized the amino groups must be removed. This reaction of deaminization occurs in several steps and in many of the tissues of the body but primarily in the liver and kidney. The amino group that is removed forms ammonia before it is converted to *urea* in order to be excreted from the body. The urea, which is the major nitrogenous product in the decomposition of proteins in the body, is then carried to the kidneys where it is eliminated in the urine. The oxidation of the remainder of the amino acid, however, follows the pathway of carbohydrate metabolism (Fig. 5.10). After the amino acids have been oxidized for energy, the end products are excreted from the body as carbon dioxide, water, urea, and other nitrogenous constituents. The kidneys are the pathway of excretion of the nitrogenous end products of protein metabolism.

Conversion of Amino Acids to Carbohydrate and Fat: As has been noted in the discussion of carbohydrate and fat metabolism, amino acids may be converted to either carbohydrate or fat in the normal processes of metabolism (Fig. 5.10).

Some Disorders that may Interfere with Metabolism

Disorders may occur caused by faulty metabolism of the food nutrients. These disorders which are related to heredity are now referred to as *inborn errors of metabolism*. Diabetes mellitus is the most common one; others, phenylketonuria and galactosemia, occur less frequently.

Diabetes Mellitus: Diabetes mellitus, which is estimated to affect more than two million people in the United States alone, is caused by the inability of the pancreatic cells to produce sufficient insulin to oxidize and store body glucose (Fig. 5.9). The characteristic symptoms of diabetes are excessive hunger, thirst, and urine output; accumulation of organic acids and acetone in the blood; weakness; and loss of body weight. With adequate treatment even severe diabetics are able to carry on active, productive lives.

The treatment of diabetes consists essentially of adjusting the patient's diet to his limited supply of endogenous insulin. In general the type of diet recommended contains approximately 40% of the total Calories as carbohydrate, 45% as fat, and 15% as protein. If, however, the supply of endogenous insulin is markedly insufficient for dietary control, insulin then must be administered hypodermically. Oral hypoglycemic agents have been developed that sometimes aid in the control of diabetes. "Orinase" and "Diabinese" are two of the oral hypoglycemic agents now used.

Other Inborn Errors of Metabolism: At the present time over fifty inborn errors of metabolism have been identified. They are all transmitted in a hereditary manner, caused by an abnormality in one or more of the genes, and all are rare. These disorders have been found to involve the metabolism of carbohydrates, lipids, amino acids, purines, pyrimidines, and minerals as well as defects in the renal tubular transport, and blood and blood-forming tissues. The expression of the metabolic error may vary from no symptoms whatsoever, as in the case of pentosuria, to the severe symptoms encountered in phenylketonuria or galactosemia. The therapy for the control of these metabolism anomalies may involve dietary measures or pharmaceutical agents, depending upon the nature of the disorders.

To illustrate the different kinds of inborn errors of metabolism, a brief description of a carbohydrate defect, a mineral defect, and two amino acid defects are presented here. For a more comprehensive review of inborn errors of metabolism, however, the paper by Sinclair is suggested.

Galactosemia is a disorder resulting from the deficiency of specific enzyme (galactose-I-phosphate-uridyl-transferase) involved in the conversion of galactose to glucose. This disorder, which usually manifests itself shortly after birth, results in failure to thrive, enlargement of the liver, galactose in the urine, jaundice, cataracts, and mental retardation. A restricted intake of foods containing lactose is the treatment now described for galactosemia. It has been observed that although diet therapy did not appear to improve the cataracts of galactosemia, children whose diets were vigorously restricted in lactose were more intelligent than those whose diets were restricted little or not at all.

Wilson's disease is a metabolic error associated with a disturbance in copper metabolism characterized by an enzymatic deficiency in the production of the copper protein ceruloplasmin. In this disorder, copper deposition occurs in the brain, liver, and other organs with the result that the normal function of the cells is inhibited. An oral therapeutical agent penicillamine, is now used to accelerate the removal of the excess copper from the body.

Phenylketonuria is an inborn error of metabolism that develops soon after birth and involves a deficiency of an enzyme in the liver necessary for the conversion of the amino acid, phenylalanine, to another amino acid, tyrosine. Motor disorders, eczema, sometimes fair skin and hair, musty-smelling urine, and mental retardation are some of the typical symptoms of this disorder. A restricted intake of foods containing phenylalanine is used to control this disorder. Because phenylalanine is widespread in all protein foods, synthetic amino acid products low in the amino acid ("Ketonil" and "Lofenalac") have been developed to treat the PKU patient. The improvement of the mental retardation in PKU children is apparently related to the early use of the restricted diet. There is some evidence that dietary treatment of phenylketonuria can be relaxed in the early school years of the patient.

Histidinemia, an inborn error of metabolism that involves a deficiency of the enzyme, histidase, which catalyzes the transfer of the amino acid, histidine, to urocanic acid was first described in 1962. In the five known cases of histidinemia, the only serious clinical manifestation of the disorder appears to a speech defect; none are mentally retarded.

6

Need for Energy

6.1. Introduction

In the previous chapters it has been studied that any or all of the food stuffs such as carbohydrates, proteins, amino acids etc. may be utilized as fuel for muscular work. The body is not restricted to any are kind of food stuff for the support of any one kind of work but has very great power of converting one nutrient into, of use it in place of , another. The carbohydrates, proteins and fats are the major constituents of food that supply energy to the body since the most conspicuous nutritive requirement is that of energy for the work of the body and since carbohydrates, fats, proteins etc. serve as fuel to yield energy, one basis of comparison is that of every value.

The amount of carbohydrate, fats and protein in a food determines its energy value. The source of energy in these compounds is energy from sunlight. The plants utilize this solar energy and convert it into food by the process of photosynthesis. Animals are dependent on food as the source of energy to do work and maintain body temperature. Thus the process of photosynthesis is basic to life itself.

This potential energy stored in food is released and combustion, when these compounds (carbohydrates, fats, proteins) are burnt in the laboratory or oxidized in the body, energy is released through a series of steps or a series of reactions. Organic compounds are combustible where as inorganic compounds are non-combustible and so H_2O (water) which is an inorganic compound has no fuel value.

Foods with relatively large proportions of carbohydrate, fat, and protein per unit of weight are high in energy content (caloric value) whereas those with small proportions are low in caloric value. An ordinary pat of butter has an energy value of 50 Cal. because of its high fat content. In contrast, the portion of tomato juice equivalent to the energy value (in Calories) of the pat of butter is 35 times greater by weight, or one cup.

Since the body does not make any great distinction among the foodstuffs as sources of energy. The fuel value of the diet as a whole is utilized to meet the energy requirements of the whole body. For the present, therefore, it is the fuel value of the day's dietary which we have to consider rather than the distribution of this as regards protein, fat and carbohydrate.

The total food (or energy) requirement is best expressed in Calories per day, either for the whole body or per kilogram of body weight, and for convenience of discussion it is usually assumed that the average body weight (without clothing) is for men 70 kilograms (154 pounds) and for women eight tenths as much, 56 kilograms (123 pounds).

6.2. Factors which Determine the Total Energy Need

The three main factors that determine the total energy need of an individual are the *basal metabolism*, the *physical activity*, and the *specific dynamic effect of food.* The basal metabolism, generally represents the largest fraction of the total energy expenditure. It is the minimum amount of energy required to carry on the vital life processes of the body when awake. The *regulation of body temperature* is an important entity in the basal metabolism. Energy for the performance of all types of physical activity ranks next to basal metabolism in amount of energy expended. The extra energy needed to metabolize food (with a resulting increase in heat production, which is known as the specific dynamic effect) is the third factor that is part of the total energy requirement. This third factor is a small one.

6.3. Definition of Terms

Some of the specific terms used in the study of energy metabolism are *calorie, calorimetry*, and *calorimeter.*

A *calorie* is the standard unit used to measure energy. The calorie used in nutrition is called the kilocalorie or large calorie and is written with a capital letter (Calorie or Cal.). This unit is one thousand times greater than the small calorie (calorie or cal.) used in chemistry or physics. To distinguish between the size of the large and small calorie, the example of the energy value of a pat of butter is cited. A pat of butter contains 50 Cal. or 50,000 cal. Although the word "Calorie" is often used to describe the potential energy in food, it is not a nutrient but rather a unit of measure of heat.

Calorimetry is the measurement of the amount of heat given off or absorbed. The energy value of particular food and the daily energy needs of a person are both determined by calorimetry, and expressed in terms of Calories. If the measurement is made from the actual heat produced, this referred to as *direct calorimetry.* However, of the amount of oxygen consumed and/ or the carbon dioxide produced is used as a basis to indirectly measure heat production, this is known as *indirect calorimetry.*

A *calorimeter* is an instrument or apparatus that is used to measure the calories of heat produced. The energy value of foods is measured by either the oxy- or bomb calorimeter. The instruments used to measure the heat production of man,directly or indirectly, are the Armsby Calorimeter and the Benedict-Roth apparatus.

6.4. Methods of Studying Food Requirements of Man

The four important methods of studying the food requirements of man are as follows:

(1) By observing the amount of food consumed (*dietary studies*).
(2) By observing the amount of oxygen consumed, or carbon dioxide produced, or both (*respiration experiments*).
(3) By determining the balance of intake and output (*carbon and nitrogen balance experiments*).
(4) By direct measurement of heat given off by the body (*calorimeter experiments*).

1. Dietary Studies

From most of the dietary studies we get only a general indication of the food habits of the people; but in cases where person have maintained for a long time the same dietary habits and other conditions of life, and the body weight has remained practically constant, it can be assumed that the food has furnished just the right quantity of energy for the maintenance of the body under the observed conditions.

Great care must be taken in drawing inferences from the body weight because of the readiness with which the body gains or loses moisture. Athletes often lose 2 or 3 pounds in an hour of vigorous exercise, and regain it, through food and drink, in less than a day. Gain or loss of body weight during short periods, therefore, does not by any means necessarily imply a corresponding gain or loss of fat. When, however, the weight remain nearly the same for months at a time, it can be assumed that there is no important gain or loss of tissue and that the body is receiving just the proper total amount of food for its needs. Under these conditions an accurate observation of the food consumed may give indications about the actual food requirement. Of such dietary studies perhaps the most useful individual example is that of Neumann, who reduced his diet to what appeared to be just about sufficient for his needs and then recorded all food and drink taken during a period of 10 months in which the body weight remained nearly constant. The average daily food furnished:

Table. 6.1 Data of Neumann's First Dietary Study

Nutrients	*Weight*	*Factors*		*Calories*	*Total Calories per day*
Protein	66.1 grams	× 4.	=	264.4	
Fat	83.5 grams	× 9.	=	751.5	2242
Carbohydrate	306.5 grams	× 4.	=	1226.0	

The 2242 Calories per day were thus fully sufficient to meet the energy requirements of this man, whose weight was 66.5 to 67 kilograms (about 147 pounds) and who was engaged at his usual (mainly sedentary) professional work in the Hygienic Institute at Kiel.

Later, when his weight had increased to 71.5 kilograms (157 pounds) because of following for a time a more liberal diet (furnishing about 2600 Calories per day), he took up his second dietary study which was continued for 8 months, during which the average daily food consumption was found to be as follows:

Table.6.1. Data of Neumann's Second Dietary Study

Nutrients	*Weight*	*Factors*		*Calories*	*Total Calories per day*
Protein	76.2 grams	× 4.	=	304.8	
Fat	109.0 grams	× 9.	=	981.0	2000
Carbohydrate	178.6 grams	× 4.	=	714.4	

The body weight remained nearly constant.

From these studies it was inferred that a man of average size, living a normal professional life involving no manual labour in the ordinary sense, but not excluding such muscular movements as are naturally incidental to a sedentary occupation, found his energy requirements satisfied with food furnishing 2000 to 2250 Calories per day.

2. Respiration Experiments

As the foodstuffs provide energy through their oxidations in the body, it is evident that a measure of the energy metabolism can be obtained by finding either the amount of foodstuffs oxidized or the amount of oxygen which is consumed in the process. The apparatus devised and used by Zuntz for this purpose provides a mask, fitting air tight over the mouth and nose and connected by means of valved pipes with apparatus for measuring and analyzing the inspired and expired air. With its help one can determine the volume of oxygen entering, and the volume leaving, the lungs. The difference is the volume consumed in the body.

Benedict devised an improved form of respiration apparatus. In his apparatus the subject breathes, either through a mouth- or nose-piece, from a current of air which is purified and kept in circulation in the same way as that of the respiration calorimeter chamber. The carbon dioxide which the man produces is absorbed quantitatively and the oxygen which he consumes is measured by the change in level of a spirometer previously filled with oxygen gas which drops as oxygen is consumed by the man.

A given volume of oxygen used in the body may liberate somewhat different amounts of heat, according as it oxidizes fat, carbohydrate, or protein. For accurate estimations of the energy liberated it is thus necessary to know the kind of material oxidized, as also the amount of oxygen consumed. This is calculated from the respiratory quotient.

As the amount of protein broken down in the body can be estimated from the nitrogen excretion, the determination of the respiratory quotient along with the oxygen consumption shows the extent of the combustion in the body and the proportions of fat and carbohydrate burned. These data can be used to calculate the energy.

Actually it is not necessary to go through the actual calculation of the amounts of fat and carbohydrate burned, since the energy derived from a liter of oxygen when used to burn carbohydrate and fat in different proportions can be calculated once for all and expressed in relation to the respiratory quotient as shown in Table 6.3.

It is then only necessary to determine the respiratory quotient, or if working under conditions for which it is known, the volume of oxygen consumed so as, to know the number of Calories of energy metabolized. This is known as the method of *indirect calorimetry.*

This method of studying the energy metabolism allows experiments being carried out quickly, and is thus useful for the direct investigation of conditions which affect energy metabolism, such as muscular work or the eating of food. The periods of observation cannot be very long, but the probable results for the 24 hours' metabolism can be estimated by the data obtained during frequent short periods at different times of the day and night.

From the results of various observations made by the Zuntz method, Magnus-Levy estimated the minimum metabolism of a man of average size kept absolutely motionless and fasting at 1625 Calories per day. Food barely sufficient for maintenance would increase this by 175 Calories, and such incidental muscular movements as would ordinarily be made by a man at rest in bed would involve another 200, making a total of 2000 Calories as the estimated food requirement of a man at rest with a maintenance diet. Magnus-Levy further estimated that the man, if doing no work (in the ordinary sense), but allowed to move about the room instead of remaining in bed, would require 2230 Calories per day.

3. Carbon and Nitrogen Balance Experiments

By comparing the constituents of the food consumed ("intake") and of the substances eliminated from the body ("output"), the

Table 6.3. Energy Values of Oxygen and Carbon Dioxide at Different Respiratory Quotients (Zuntz and Schumburg)

Respiratory Quotient	*Calories Per Liter of Oxygen*	*Calories Per Liter of Carbon Dioxide*	*Calories Per Gram of Carbon Dioxide*
0.70	4.686	6.694	3.408
0.71	4.690	6.606	3.363
0.72	4.702	6.531	3.325
0.73	4.714	6.458	3.288
0.74	4.727	6.388	3.252
0.75	4.739	6.319	3.217
0.76	4.752	6.253	3.183
0.77	4.764	6.187	3.150
0.78	4.776	6.123	3.117
0.79	4.789	6.062	3.086
0.80	4.801	6.001	3.055
0.81	4.813	5.942	3.025
0.82	4.825	5.884	2.996
0.83	4.838	5.829	2.967
0.84	4.850	5.774	2.939
0.85	4.863	5.721	2.912
0.86	4.875	5.669	2.886
0.87	4.887	5.617	2.860
0.88	4.900	5.568	2.835
0.89	4.912	5.519	2.810
0.90	4.924	5.471	2.785
0.91	4.936	5.424	2.761
0.92	4.948	5.378	2.738
0.93	4.960	5.333	2.715
0.94	4.973	5.290	2.693
0.95	4.985	5.247	2.671
0.96	4.997	5.205	2.650
0.97	5.010	5.165	2.629
0.98	5.022	5.124	2.609
0.99	5.034	5.085	2.589
1.00	5.047	5.047	2.569

material actually oxidized and the energy liberated in the oxidation can be determined.

The intake is found by weighing and analyzing all food eaten; the output by collecting and determining the end products eliminated through the lungs, the kidneys, the intestines, and also through the skin. The time unit in experiments upon the intake and output is almost always 24 hours, the experimental day beginning preferably just before breakfast. The feces belonging to the experimental days are marked, generally by giving a small amount of lampblack with the food as in ordinary digestion experiments, separated and analyzed. The end products given off by the lungs and kidneys during an experimental day are taken as measuring the material broken down in the body during the same period.

Sometime is of course needed for the elimination of the nitrogenous end products through the kidneys. The unaviodable "lag" in the elimination of nitrogen may introduce an error in interpreting the nitrogen balance unless the subject has been kept for a few days in advance upon the same diet which is to be used in the experiment.

Assuming that the total nitrogen and carbon of the absorbed food existed in the form of protein, fat, and carbohydrate, and that the amount of carbohydrate in the body is the same at the beginning and end of each experiment, it is only necessary to determine the carbon dioxide of the expired air and the carbon and nitrogen of the waste products so as to find out the quantities of material oxidized and of energy liberated in the body. Experiments of this type have played an important part in the development of our knowledge of nutrition. The calculations are usually based on the average analyses of protein and body fat. See Table 6.4.

Table 6.4. Average Elementary Composition of Protein and Fat

	Protein	*Fat*
Carbon	53	76.5
Nitrogen	16	–
Hydrogen	7	12
Oxygen	23	11.5
Sulfur	1	–
	100	100

The data of Table 6.5 were obtained with a man on ordinary mixed diet.

Table 6.5 Calculation of Energy Metabolism from Carbon and Nitrogen Balances. Man of 64 Kilograms at Rest in at Water Respiration Apparatus

Intake	*Grams Per Day*				
	Protein	*Fat*	*Carbo-hydrate*	*Nitrogen*	*Carbon*
Total in food	94.4	82.5	289.8	15.1	239.0
Lost in digestion	5.4	3.7	3.2	0.9	7.4
Absorbed	89.0	78.8	286.6	14.2	231.6
Output					
By lungs					207.3
By kidneys				16.2	12.2
Metabolized				16.2	219.5
Balance				–2.0	+12.1

A loss of 2.0 grams of body nitrogen shows that (2.0 × 6.25 =) 12.5 grams of body protein has been burned. Also there were 89.0 grams absorbed from food, and , therefore, in all 101.5 grams of total protein burned.

The amount of carbohydrate burned was taken to be the same as that absorbed from the food, viz 286.6 grams per day.

From the carbon balance and the above data, therefore, we estimate the amount of fat burned as under:

12.5 grams body protein yield (12.5 × 53 % =)	6.6 grams carbon
and there were in the absorbed food	231.6 grams carbon
∴ total available was	238.2 grams carbon
But total catabolized was only	219.5 grams carbon
∴ the body stored in the form of fat	18.7 grams carbon

Since fat contains 76.5 % carbon, 1 gram carbon = 1.307 grams fat.

∴ 18.7 grams carbon =	24.4 grams fat.		
The body therefore absorbed	78.8 grams fat		
stored	24.4 grams fat		
burned	54.4 grams fat		

In all, the body burned per day		
101.5 grams protein, yielding	$(101.5 \times 4.35 =)$	442 Calories
54.4 grams fat, yielding	$(54.4 \times 9.45 =)$	515 Calories
286.6 grams carbohydrate, yielding	$(286.6 \times 4.1 =)$	1175 Calories
		2132 Calories

By means of the carbon and nitrogen balance, Sonden and Tigerstedt studied the energy metabolism of eight resting men between nineteen and forty-four years of age, with results which varied for the different subjects from 1853 to 2292 Calories per day. Many other experimenters have used the same method with similar results.

4. Calorimeter Experiments

It is the most direct, and also most convincing, way of ascertaining the energy metabolism. *This method of direct calorimetry* consists in measuring the total energy expenditure of the body as heat or as heat or as heat and mechanical work by confining the subject in a chamber allowing of actual measurement of the heat produced. It was only after the development of the Atwater-rosa-Benedict respiration calorimeter that complete and satisfactory data covering periods of one to several days were obtained. This apparatus consisted of an air- tight copper chamber. surrounded by zinc and wooden walls with air-spaces between, and was large enough for a man to live in without discomfort, being about 7 feet long, 4 feet wide, and $6\frac{1}{2}$ feet high. An opening in the front of the apparatus, that was sealed with a pane of glass during an experiment, acted as both door and window, admitting sufficient light for reading and writing. A smaller opening, having tightly fitting caps on both ends, was used for passing food, drink, excreta, etc., into and out of the chamber. The chamber was furnished with a folding bed, chair, and table and was ventilated by means of a current of air. The carbon dioxide and water given off by the subject being removed by circulating the air through purifying apparatus

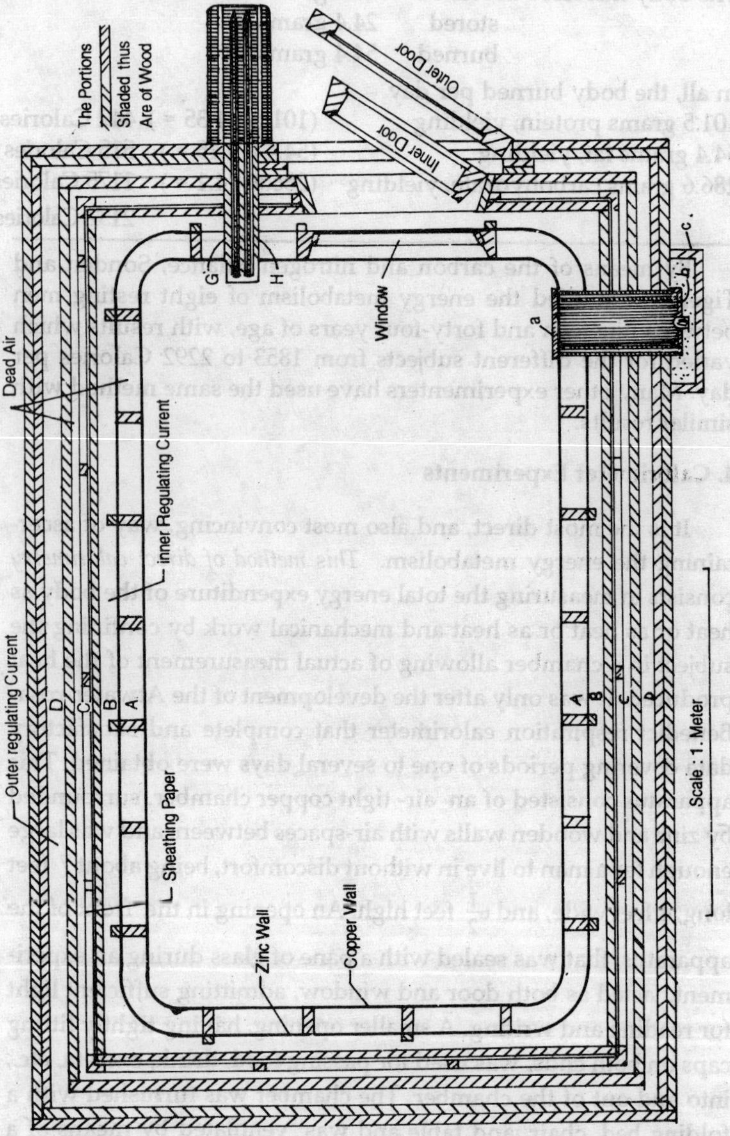

Fig. 6.1. Horizontal section of the original Atwater-Rose-Benedict respiration calorimeter.

and the oxygen which the subject used being replaced by adding weighed amounts of oxygen to the air current as required. In this way it is possible to carry out, in the calorimeter, metabolism experiments in which the oxygen and hydrogen as also the carbon and nitrogen balances are determined, and from these data the gain or loss of carbohydrate as also of protein and fat can be measured.

The ventilating air current is regulated in such a way that it enters and leaves the calorimeter at the same temperature and between the copper and zinc walls are placed a large number of thermo-electric junctions connected with a delicate galvanometer by means of which each wall is tested every four minutes, day and night, during the progress of an experiment, and the mere traces of heat that may pass to or from the calorimeter through its walls are quickly detected and made to balance each other. Thus there is no gain or loss of heat either through the walls of the chamber or by the ventilating air current, and the heat given off by the subject can leave only by the means particularly provided for carrying it out and measuring it. A part of the heat liberated is carried from the chamber in latent form by the water vapor in the outgoing air, which is accurately determined. The remaining heat is brought away by means of a current of cold water circulating through a copper pipe coiled near the ceiling of the chamber. The quantity of water that passes through the pipe and the difference between the temperature at which it enters and that at which it leaves the coil are carefully determined and show how much heat is thus brought out of the chamber.

In recent years several different forms of respiration apparatus and calorimeters, based on these principles but adapted in size and shape to different types of experimentation, have come into use.

In 1913 Armsby compiled a summary of experiments upon men, dogs, and cattle which showed that the difference between the total heat production as computed and as directly measured was only one fourth of one per cent, or quite within the limits of accuracy of experimental methods of this sort.

Since the time of Armsby's compilation, the agreement between the observed and computed heat production has been confirmed in many additional experiments, both by the same and different experimenters.

Summary of the Evidence Obtained by the Different Methods

Results obtained by all four of the methods described are found to be strikingly consistent and so leads to the conclusion that the food requirements of a young to middle-aged man of average size, without muscular work, eating a mixed diet sufficient to meet his need, approximates 2000 Calories per day, and that such muscular activity as is incidental to very quiet living indoors may be expected to raise this requirement to about 2200 Calories per day.

Lusk summarized the mean energy requirement of an averagesized man in somewhat more precise terms as follows: Absolute rest in bed without food, 1680 Calories; Absolute rest in bed with food, 1840 Calories; Rest in bed 8 hours, sitting in chair 16 hours, with food, 2168 Calories.

7

The Energy Value of Foods

7.1. Introduction

The amount of carbohydrate, fat and protein in a food determines its energy value. The energy value of food is generally expressed in nutrition in terms of *kilocaloric* and traditionally designated the *large calorie.* The trend, however is slowly moving away from the use of the term calorie towards the more accurate practice of calling the kilo calorie by its own name.

7.2. Heats of Combustion of the Food Stuffs and Its Determination

The *calorific value* or heat of combustion of any substance is the quantity of energy liberated by burning a given quantity of the combustible material.

Determination of Calorific Value of Food

To determine the calorific value of a food stuff we use *(i) a bomb calorimeter* or *(ii) the oxycalorimeter.*

Bomb Calorimeter Method

In its original form it was devised by Bertholet. The Bertholet Bomb which was most used in the quantitative development of the fundamental energy relations of food materials and physiological products was devised by Atwater and Blakeslee. It consists of a heavy steel bomb, A, with a platinum or gold plated copper lining and a cover held tightly in place by means of a strong screw collar (Fig. 7.1).

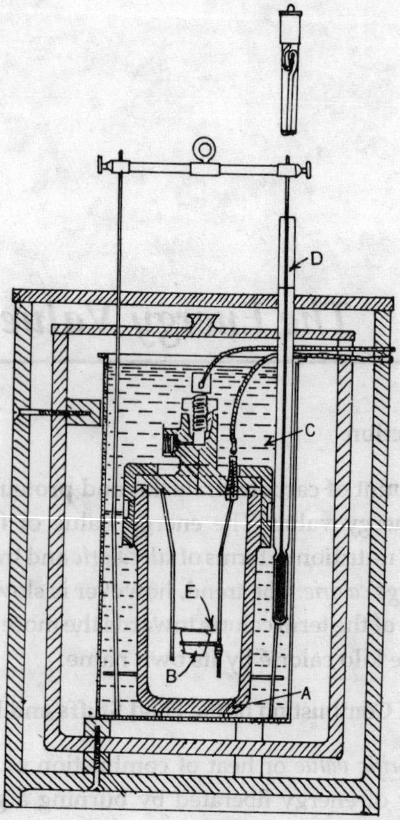

Fig 7.1. The Atwater bomb calorimeter.

A weighed quantity of the given food sample, generally pressed into pellets, is placed in a capsule, B, with in the bomb. It is then closed except for the oxygen value, charged with oxygen to a pressure of a minimum of 20 atmospheres (300 lbs/sq. inch). The oxygen valve is then closed and the bomb immersed in a weighed amount of water, C. The water is constantly stirred and its temperature noted at intervals of one minute with the help of a differential thermometer, D, capable of being read to one thousandth of a degree. After the rate at which the temperature of the water rises or falls has been determined, the sample is ignited by means of an electric fuse, E, and as a result of large amount of oxygen present it undergoes rapid and complete combustion. The heat liberated is passed to the water in which the bomb is immersed, and the resulting rise in temperature is determined. The thermometer readings are also continued through an "after period," so that the "radiation correction" may be calculated and the observed rise of temperature corrected accordingly. This corrected rise, multiplied by the total heat capacity of the apparatus and the water in which it is immersed, shows the total heat liberated in the bomb. From this must be deducted the heat arising from accessory combustion (the oxidation of the iron wire used as a fuse, etc.) to obtain the number of Calories arising from the combustion of the sample.

If we use a*diabatic form* of bomb calorimeter (which is most commonly used these days) there is no need to make corrections for heat losses.

Another apparatus used to determine the energy value of food is the *oxy-calorimeter.* It was devised by Benedict and coworkers. It measures the volume of oxygen needed to burn a known weight of the food. From this, by means of factors established by use of the bomb calorimeter, the calorific value of the food is calculated.

The bomb calorimeter measures the heat produced when a food is actually burned where as the oxy calorimeter measures the oxygen used and carbon dioxide produced during the burning of a food.

The heats of combustion of individual carbohydrates, fats, proteins differ some what, (e.g. the energy yield of sucrose is 3.96 k col/g and that of starch is 4.23 k col/g, of butter fat it is 9.21 but of lard (a fat) it is 9.48 k cal/g, for practical use there have been averaged as follows:

Carbohydrates	4.15 k cal/g
Fats	9.40 k cal/g
Proteins	5.65 k cal/g

The energy values of the food stuffs do not represent the energy actually available to body cells.

When heat of combustion is corrected for losses in digestion and for unmetabolized urinary substances, energy value of foods is designated.

Available Energy or Physiological Fuel Value

The Available energy of the major food stuffs is as follows (Fig 7.2):

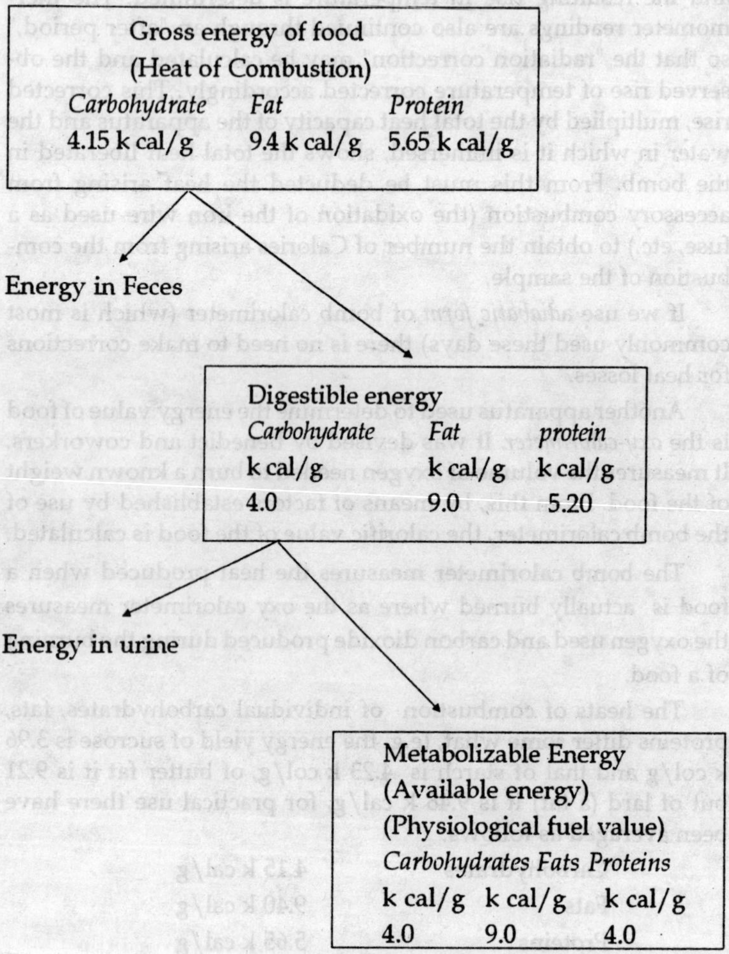

Fig.7.2. Energy Value of Food.

The terms digestible energy and metabolizable energy are more accurately designated *apparent digestible energy and apparent metbolizable energy.*

Table 7.1. gives heats of combustion of same pounds.

Table 7.1. Heats of Combustion and Elementary Composition of Typical Compounds

Substance	*Heat of Combustion Calories per Gram*
Glucose	3.75
Sucrose	3.96
Starch } Glycogen }	4.22
Body fat	9.60
Butter fat	9.30
Edestin	5.64
Legumin	5.62
Gliadin	5.74
Casein	5.85
Albumin	5.80
Gelatin	5.30
Creatinine	4.58
Urea	2.53

The physiological Fuel Values as calculated for carbohydrates, Fats and Protein are shown in Table 7.2.

Table 7.2

	Carbo-hydrates kcal/g	*Fats kcal/g*	Proteins kcal/g
Fuel values	4.10	9.45	5.65
Less due to in complete combustion of nitrogen	—	—	–1.25
% age of digestibility	4.10 × 0.98	9.45 × 0.95	4.40 × 0.92
Physiological fuel value	4	9	4

These values have been calculated on the basis of the fact that 1.25 k cal/g is the energy lost due to incomplete combustion of nitrogen and that only 98%, 95% and 92% of carbohydrate, fat and protein ingested is absorbed by the human digestive mechanism.

Table 7.3. Physiological Energy Factors more Specific than those of Atwater

Food or Food Group	*Protein Cal. per Gm*	*Fat Cal .per Gm.*	*Carbohydrate (by difference) Cal .per Gm.*
1	2	3	4
Milk, milk products	4.27	8.79	3.87
Meat, fish	4.27	9.02	—
Eggs	4.36	9.02	—
Separated fats			
Butter fat	—	8.79	—
Other animal fats	—	9.02	—
Vegetable fats and oils, hydrogenated fats margarine	—	8.84	—
Cereals			
Barley, light	3.55	8.37	3.95
Cornmeal, whole ground	2.73	8.37	4.03
Cornmeal, determinated	3.46	8.37	4.16
Crackers, soda, plain	4.23	8.37	4.12
Macaroni	3.91	8.37	4.12
Noodles (with egg)	3.91	8.84	4.12
Oatmeal (rolled oats)	3.69	8.37	4.12
Rice, polished	3.78	8.37	4.12
Rye flour, whole grain	2.41	8.37	3.78
Wheat, 97-100% extraction	3.59	8.37	3.78
Wheat, 85-93% extraction	3.78	8.37	3.95
Wheat, 70-74% extraction	4.05	8.37	4.12
Other cereals, refined	3.87	8.37	4.12

(contd.)

1	2	3	4
Other foods			
Dry beans, peas, nuts	3.47	8.37	4.07
Potatoes and starchy roots	2.74	8.37	4.03
Other underground crops	2.74	8.37	3.84
Other vegetables	2.44	8.37	3.57
Fruits	3.36	8.37	3.60
Lemons, lemon juice	3.36	8.37	2.70
Sugar (disaccharide)	—	—	3.87
(glucose)	—	—	3.68

Limitations in the use of physiological Fuel Values

The physiological fuel values are not valid to use in calculating the calorie values of international food supplies as the energy value 4-9-4 if used will lead to wrong results. It is because of the fact that the physiological fuel values of 4-9-4 are applicable only to the foods of average mixed American diet and not to single foods or to foods of mixed diets eaten by other nations. To illustrate it we can table the case of the energy value of rice. According to 4-9-4 rule the average value for 100g of polished rice used in America is 35/k cal but for the same quantity of brown rice or under milled rice used in orient averages to 320 – 340 k cal respectively.

To over came such discrepancies the need was felt for a universal method for the determination and expression of food energy values.

8

The Basal Energy Metabolism and Food Requirement

8.1. Introduction

The foundations for basic principles of energy metabolism were laid by Lavoisier, who is also known as "Father of Nutrition", in the eighteenth century. The other important contributors to it are Justus von Liebig, Max Rubner, Wilbur Atwater, Henry Arwishy and many others. After World War II it became apparent that available information as the energy composition of food substances and the energy needs of mass was inadequate and it focussed the need for new energy research. There has been a of interest in energy metabolism during last 30-40 years.

8.2. Energy Needs for Basal Metabolism

The term *basal metabolism* refers to the energy metabolism of the body when at complete rest (both mentally and physically) in the so-called "post-absorptive state" (12 to 18 hours after the last previous intake of food) in a room of comfortable temperature and when the body temperature is within normal range. "If this last condition is not satisfied, the deviation from the normal temperature must be determined." This basal energy metabolism for a given age and size is used as the starting point for the calculation of the total energy requirement of individuals of different muscular activities, and also as a basis of comparison in pathological disturbances, or in studies of the influence of age, sex, race, or of previous or immediate environment.

Thus it is the amount of energy required to carry on the vital life processes of the body (the activity of heart, kidney and other organs and also the metabolic processes with in the cells) but excludes the energy required for physical activity and specific dynamic effect of food.

In a healthy adult about one-third of the basal energy is expended for functional activities of various organs. The basal metabolism determinations are used diagnosing certain disorders and diseases e.g. *hyperthyroidism* and *hypothyroidism.*

8.3. Methods of Determining Basal Metabolism

We can use the method of *direct* or *indirect calorimetry*. During these determinations it is assumed that the individual is oxidising a mixed diet.

For the determination of basal metabolism we generally use Benedict - Roth apparatus for measuring the amount of oxygen used by an individual. It is most satisfactory instrument for medical diagnosis as it requires very short time for measurement and is easy to operate.

The Tissot apparatus involves the collection and analysis of expired air of an individual, is used for determining the basal metabolism in experimental studies. This method is expensive both in operating time and cost of equipment, but because a greater accuracy in the basal measurement, it is a valuable tool in energy research. Direct calorimetry, is used most frequently in the study of energy need during exercise.

8.4. Conditions Under Which Basal Metabolism should be Measured

The basal metabolism should be measured under the following conditions:

(i) It should be made 12-18 hours after the last intake of food.

(ii) It should generally be done in mornings.

(iii) It should be done when the person under test is awake and lying quietly in a room of comfortable temperature. (During sleep there is about 10% lowering in metabolism of a person)

(iv) The person under investigation should be relaxed. (Nervousness of tensión causes an increase in the heat production).

8.5. How to Compute the Basal Metabolism

A very crude method that can be used to compute basal metabolism is as follows:-

Basal metabolism = 1 k cal × body weight in kg × 24 hour.
(in K cal/24 hours)

Thus for a college student weighing 178 lb.

it would be equal to $1 \times \frac{178}{2.2} \times 24$ [1kg =2.2 lb]

=1921 K cal/24 hours.

8.6 Factors which may Affect the Basal Metabolism

The basal metabolism is affected by *(i)* body size, *(ii)* body composition, *(iii)* age, *(iv)* health, *(v)* secretion of ductless glands, *(vi)* pregnancy, *(vii)* growth etc.

Influence of the Size, Shape and Composition of the Body Size

Numerous determinations of basal metabolic rates have been made on humans and other species. From these it has became clear that metabolic rate varies with body size. For many years however, there has been considerable discussion and disagreement in attempts to establish a constant relationship between metabolic rate and a unit of body size that would apply to large and small animals alike.

It clinical practice it is customary to express B M R in relation to surface area, that is, k cal per hour per square metre of body surface. This relationship is based on assumption that heat loss and therefore B M R are proportional to surface area. Many formulae have been proposed for calculation of body surface from weight and height. The formula of DuBois and DuBois (1916) is one that appears to be will accepted

$$A = W^{0.425} \times H^{0.725} \times 71.84$$

where A is surface area in m^2, W is weight in kg and H is height is metres.

The influence of body size an Basal metabolism was illustrated by. Taylor by using pieces of food to represent the area of body surface.

In the first example (Fig. 8.1) Blocks A and B represent two men of the same age and body weight but who are different in shape, one being tall and the other short. Even though Blocks A and B are identical in volume and weight, the surface area of Block A is about one-third greater than that of Block B. Thus the tall man will have a higher basal metabolism per unit of body weight than the shorter man of the same weight.

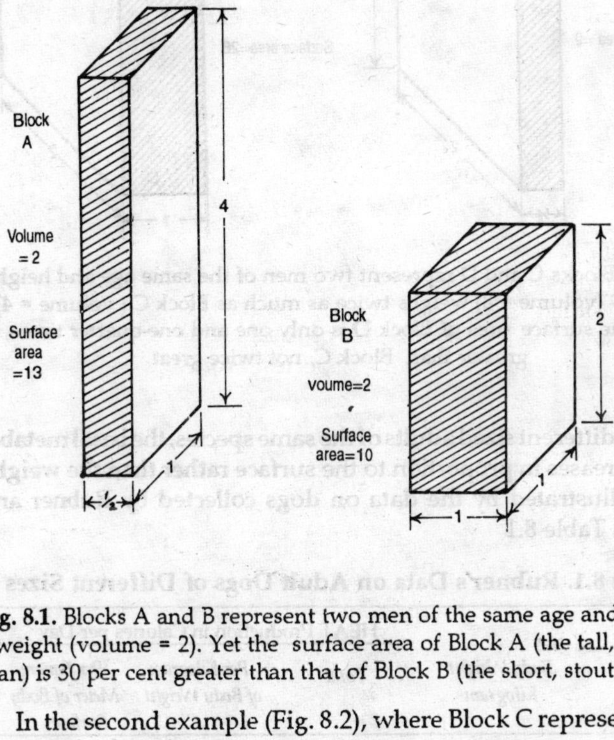

Fig. 8.1. Blocks A and B represent two men of the same age and body weight (volume = 2). Yet the surface area of Block A (the tall, thin man) is 30 per cent greater than that of Block B (the short, stout man.)

In the second example (Fig. 8.2), where Block C represents the thin man and Block D represents the stout man, the two men are of the same height and age but the thin man weighs one-half as much as the stout man. Here the surface area of the stout block is only about one and one-fourth times greater than the thin block, not twice as great. These examples serve to show the important relationship of body size and shape to the actual basal heat production of an individual.

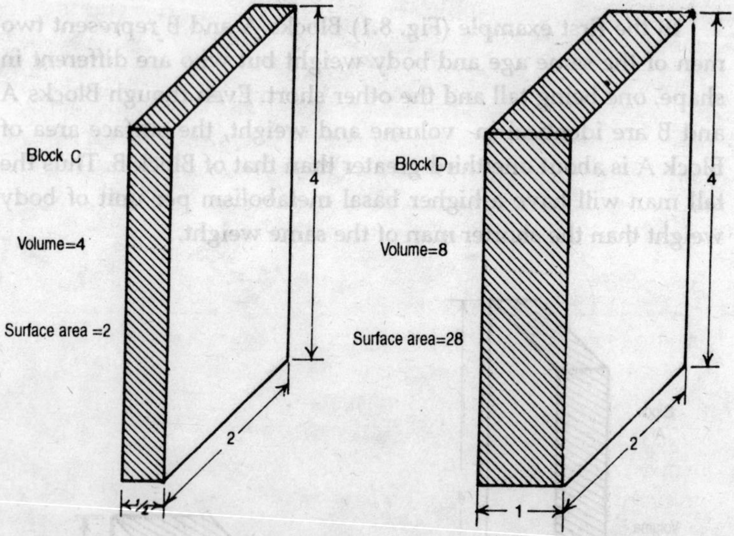

Fig.8.2. Blocks C and D represent two men of the same age and height. Block D (volume = 8) weighs twice as much as Block C (volume = 4), yet the surface area of Block D is only one and one-quarter times greater than Block C, not twice great.

For different sized adults of the same species, the basal metabolism increases in proportion to the surface rather than the weight. this is illustrated by the data on dogs collected by Rubner and listed in Table 8.1

Table 8.1. Rubner's Data on Adult Dogs of Different Sizes

No	Body Weight Kilograms	HEAT Production in Calories per Day		
		Total	Per Kilogram of Body Weight	Per Square Meter of Body Surface
I	3.10	273.6	88.25	1214
II	6.44	417.3	64.79	1120
III	9.51	619.7	65.16	1183
IV	17.70	817.7	46.20	1097
V	19.20	880.7	45.87	1207
VI	23.71	970.0	40.91	1112
VII	30.63	1124.0	36.66	1046

Here the heat production in Calories per kilogram was over twice as great in the smallest as in the largest dog, but the total metabolism was nearly proportional to the surface area throughout.

That the relationship of basal metabolism to body surface is not due simply to loss of heat through the cooling effect of the environment will be apparent from the observations upon the regulation of body temperature.

After Rubner's work it became customory to express basal energy requirements in terms of surface area than of weight. In the earlier computations the Meeh's formula was used.

$S = W^{2/3} \times C$, or $S = 12.3\sqrt[3]{W^2}$, in which *S* represents surface, *W* the weight, and the constant 12.3 represents the average value found By Meeh in a series of measurements of men.

Lissauer's modification of Meeh's formula, based on measurements of infants, is used extensively for estimating the surface area of infants and young children:

$$S = 10.3\sqrt[3]{W^2}$$

Benedict and Talbot have modified the constant of this formula to adapt it to increase in body weight up to 40 kilograms.

On the basis of their experiments DuBois and DuBois concluded that the results obtained by this formula are a bit higher. They used two methods for computing the surface.

(1) from a series of nineteen measurements of different parts of the body, the surface of each part being computed and the results added together ("linear formula"), and (2) a "height-weight formula" which they derived mathematically from the data of all available measurements of height, weight and surface.

The height-weight formula may be written thus:

$$A = W^{0.425} \times H^{0.725} \times C$$

or in the form:

$\text{Log}\, A = (\text{Log}\, W \times 0.425) + (\text{Log}\, H \times 0.725) + 1.8564$ in either of which

A = Surface area in square centimeters

H = Height in centimeters

W = Weight in kilograms

C = A constant (71. 84).

Table 8.2. Surface Area in Square meters for Different Hights and Weights

Height in centimeters	Weight in Kilograms																
	25	30	35	40	45	50	55	60	65	70	75	80	85	90	95	100	105
200							1.84	1.91	1.97	2.03	2.09	2.15	2.21	2.26	2.31	2.36	2.41
195						1.73	1.80	1.87	1.93	1.99	2.05	2.11	2.17	2.22	2.27	2.32	2.37
190				1.56	1.63	1.70	1.77	1.84	1.90	1.96	2.02	2.08	2.13	2.18	2.23	2.28	2.33
185				1.53	1.60	1.67	1.74	1.80	1.86	1.92	1.98	2.04	2.09	2.14	2.19	2.24	2.29
180				1.49	1.57	1.64	.171	1.77	1.83	1.89	1.95	2.00	2.05	2.10	2.15	2.20	2.25
175	1.19	1.28	1.36	1.46	1.53	1.60	1.67	1.73	1.79	1.85	1.91	1.96	2.01	2.06	2.11	2.16	2.21
170	1.17	1.26	1.34	1.43	1.50	1.57	1.63	1.69	1.75	1.81	1.86	1.91	1.96	2.01	2.06	2.11	
165	1.14	1.23	1.31	1.40	1.47	1.54	1.60	1.66	1.72	1.78	1.83	1.88	1.93	1.98	2.03	2.07	
160	1.12	1.21	1.29	1.37	1.44	1.50	1.56	1.62	1.68	1.73	1.78	1.83	1.88	1.93	1.98		
155	1.09	1.18	1.26	1.33	1.40	1.46	1.52	1.58	1.64	1.69	1.74	1.79	1.84	1.89			
150	1.06	1.15	1.23	1.30	1.36	1.42	1.48	1.54	1.60	1.65	1.70	1.75	1.80				
145	1.03	1.12	1.20	1.27	1.33	1.39	1.45	1.51	1.56	1.61	1.66	1.71					
140	1.00	1.09	1.17	1.24	1.30	1.36	1.42	1.47	1.52	1.57							
135	0.97	1.06	1.14	1.20	1.26	1.32	1.38	1.43	1.48								
130	0.95	1.04	1.11	1.17	1.23	1.29	1.35	1.40									
125	0.93	1.01	1.08	1.14	1.20	1.26	1.31	1.36									
120	0.91	0.98	1.04	1.10	1.16	1.22	1.27										

Using this formula DuBois and DuBois have constructed a chart from which the approximate surface area in square meters may be obtained at a glance if height and weight are known. The data given in Table 8.2. have been taken from this chart.

Differences of build (shape of body) are associated not only with varying ratios of weight to surface but also with differences of Fatness i.e. of body composition.

Types of Body Composition: The kinds of tissue that make up the body have a direct influence on the basal metabolism. In muscle tissue, for example, where oxidative processes are constantly taking place, more energy is expended than in fatty tissue. It has been estimated that an athletic-type man with well-developed muscular tissue will have a basal metabolism about 6 per cent higher than a nonathlete of comparable body surface. Men have a 5 per cent higher heat production than do women of comparable body size and age, the higher value, however, is not a sex difference, per se, but is attributed at least in part to the smaller amount of fatty tissue found in men as ***compared to women.***

Influence of Age and growth

Age: Age is still another factor which affects the basal heat production of an individual. The caloric requirement, which is based on area of body surface, reaches its highest point at about 18 months of age. Then there is a slight decrease in the caloric need from this time until the period of adolescence when another peak occurs. After the completion of growth there is a gradual decline in the basal heat production which extends from about age 20 throughout life. It has been estimated that the basal metabolism of a man at 75 years is about 20 per cent lower than that of a man at 20 years.

Climate: Living in a cold climate does not seem to affect the basal metabolism of an individual to any extent. Though nothing has yet been conclusively known about hot climate but some recent studies have pointed out that people living in tropics have lower metabolic rates. There seems to be no effect of altitude on basal metabolism.

Influence of internal secretions and pathological conditions: Some internal secretions influence the basal metabolism, specially that of the thyroid gland, thyroxine, which is quite specifically a regulator of the rate of oxidation in the body. If the thyroid gland becomes overactive, the basal metabolism increases. This increase has been known to amount to as much as 75 per cent. If, on the other hand, the activity of the thyroid is reduced, a lowering of the basal metabolism, which may amount to as much as 30%, results. Another internal secretion which affects the basal metabolism is adrenaline (adrenine, epinephrine), but its effect is much less and of much shorter duration than that of thyroxine. Overactivity of the pituitary gland tends to result in a rise of the basal metobolism, while subnormal activity may cause a fall in the basal rate. These changes are not usually of very great magnitude and are not nearly as characteristic as those due to abnormal functioning of the thyroid gland and the adrenals.

Illnesses involving an elevation of body temperature may markedly increase the basal heat production. For each degree rise in temperature above 98.6° F the basal rate is increased about 7%. For example, with a body temperature of 103.6°F, which is 5 degrees above normal, the basal metabolism will be increased 35%.

Basal metabolism is accelerated in exophthalmic goiter, leukemia, malarial and typhoid fever, and in tuberculosis accompanied by fever; it is neither increased nor decreased materially in adolescent goiter, tuberculosis unaccompanied by fever, uncomplicated cases of obesity, arthritis, gout, nephritis, and cardiac and renal disorders.

Pregnancy and Growth: The increase in total active tissue during pregnancy and growth results in an increase in the basal metabolic rate. Comparisons of the metabolic rates of pregnant woman just before delivery showed increases of 15 to 23% above their pre-pregnant rates. The additional active tissue is accounted for by the developing fetus and enlargement of certain maternal tissues. Indications are that lactation, however, does not cause an increase in the basal heat production.

Periods of rapid growth are associated with an increase in the basal metabolism. The period of most rapid growth in childhood is in infancy; a baby during the first 6 months of life will double his birth weight, and triple it by the end of 12 months. At the end of the second year of life or the early part of the third, the basal rate per square meter of body surface is the highest in the lifetime of an individual. At adolescence, when the growth rate again speeds up markedly, the basal metabolic rate increases also.

8.7 The Regulation of Body Temperature

Our body maintains its normal temperature (98.6° F) with the help of both physical and chemical means. Climate, season, housing clothing etc. affect energy metabolism mainly through their bearing upon the regulation of body temperature. It is clear that the maintenance of the body at a temperature above that of its ordinary environment involves a continual output of heat. This output of heat can be regulated in either of two ways: (1) By variations in the quantity of blood brought to the skin, which tend to control the loss of heat by radiation, conduction, and sweating; this is known as "physical regulation." (2) By an increase in the rate of oxidation in the body in response to the stimulus of external cold; such a charge in the rate of oxidation is known as "chemical regulation." The extra heat production which follows the taking of food (the specific dynamic action of the foodstuffs) may take the place of the "chemical regulation" and so help to protect the body from the necessity of burning material simply for the maintenance of its temperature. Muscular work, by increasing the production of heat in the body, may also render chemical regulation unnecessary; but apparently the specific dynamic action does not furnish energy which can be utilized for muscular work.

In general it seems probable that people wormly clothed and living in house which are heated in winter are not called upon to exercise "chemical regulation" to any considerable extent, the heat required for the maintenance of body temperature being obtained in connection with the metabolism which is essential to the maintenance of the muscular tension and the various other forms of internal work. If, however, the body be exposed to cold, it may be forced to employ "chemical regulation" with a resulting increase of the food requirement, and this will occur more readily in a thin person than in one who is well protected by subcutaneous fat.

To a large extent therefore the regulation of body temperature, in case of exposure to cold, is accomplished through the activity and tension of the muscles.

8.8. The Specific Dynamic Action of Food-stuffs

The increased heat production brought about by the ingestion of food itself is called the *specific dynamic effect.*

Determination of basal metabolic rate requires that the subject be in the postabsorptive state, that is, without food for at least 12 hours prior to the test. The reason for with holding food is that following ingestion of food, heat production increases above the resting state. This effect was first recognized by Rubber in 1902 and was called the *specific dynamic effect* of food.

In Lavoisier's experiment when food stuffs were fed individually, the increase in heat production following ingestion of protein was observed to be considerably greater than that of carbohydrate or fat.

The extra heat production following ingestion of food is known as *specific dynamic action* (SDA) of food. Some authors use the term calorigesnic effect for it.

Terroine and Bonnet (1926) attributed the high heat increment of protein to the quantity of amino nitrogen ingested and, more specifically, to the amount of amino nitrogen deaminated, that is urinary nitrogen. Borsook and Winegarden (1931) reported a positive correlation between the metabolic rate and urinary nitrogen.

Kreb (1964) proposed a theory relating calorigenic effect to the energy requirement for synthesis of ATP.

Calorigenic effect represents the additional calories necessary for ATP formation when protein rather than carbohydrate or fat serves as oxidative substrate.

8.9. The Total Caloric Requirements

For an individual it in cludes the energy expenditure for basal heat production, for physical activity and for the specific dynamic effect of the food eaten. We can estimate these either by using factorial method of calculations or by use of tables of recommended energy allowances.

The Factorial Method

In this, the caloric need is calculated from the individuals basal metabolism, his physical activity and the specific dynamic effect of his food.

Calculations for Basal Metabolism

For this we use the formula

Basal metabolism = kg of body weight × 1 k cal per hour × 24 hour

Since the basal metabolic rate is lower during sleep necessary correction is then made for hours of sleep. For this correction we use the formula

Correction for sleep = 0.1 k Cal × kg of body weight × number of hours of sleep.

This has to be subtracted from calculated basal metabolism for a 24 hour period.

Calculation for Physical Activity

The major difficulties in these calculations are *(i)* it is difficult to determine accurately the amount of time spent in any activity, and *(ii)* availability of only a limited data on the caloric expenditure for different kinds and intensities of activities.

With the development and use of respiratory gasmeter this limitation has been over come to a certain extent.

Estimate of Specific Dynamic Effect of Food Eaten

Now it is accepted practice to allot between 6-8% of the sum of energy expenditure of basal metabolism and physical activities for this factor.

The Daily Total Energy Expenditure as Estimated by Factorial Method

The calculation here is for a body weighing 154 pounds ($\frac{154}{2.2}$ kg).

Energy for Basal Metabolism = $\frac{154}{2.2} \times 1 \times 24$

=1680 k Cal/24 hours.

Correction for sleep = 0.1 × 70 × 8 (sleeps for 8 hours

=56 k Cal. in 24 hours)

Caloric expenditure for physical activities =2800 k Cal.

The allowance for specific dynamic Effect = 0.06 × [2800 + 1624]

= 265 k Cal.

Thus the total Energy Expenditure is equal to

(1680–56) + 2800+265 = 4689 k Cal.

In these calculations the calorific expenditure for the physical activities of a 70 kg college student has been evaluated on the basis of the following Tables 8.3, 8.4:

Table 8.3. A List of Students Activity for a 7-day period

	Time per Week		
Sleep	*56 hr*	*0 min*	
Washing and dressing	7	30	450 min
Washing and shaving	1	48	108
Showering	2	20	140
Eating meals and snacks	14	50	890
Sitting in classes	20	0	1200
Standing in chemistry lab	6	0	360
Running with the track team	6	25	385
Swimming (pleasure)	0	50	50
Studying, sitting reading	19	20	1160
Studying, sitting writing	10	20	620
Walking (about 2.27 mph)	10	15	615
Walking rapidly (5,80 mph)	0	10	10
Driving an automobile	10	0	600
Attending a movie	2	12	132
	168	0	

Table 8.4. Expenditure of Energy For Various Activities

	Energy Cost of Activity k Cal./kg/min	*Time Spent min*	*Energy Expended k Cal./kg*
Washing and dressing	0.0382	450	17.19
Washing and shaving	0.0419	108	4.53
Showering	0.0466	140	6.52
Eating meals and snacks	0.0204	890	18.16
Sitting in classes	0.0245	1200	29.40
Standing in chemistry lab	0.0356	360	12.82
Running with the track team	0.2203	385	84.82
Swimming (pleasure)	0.1454	50	7.27
Studying, sitting reading	0.0176	1160	20.42
Studying, sitting writing	0.0268	620	16.62
Walking (about 2.27 mph)	0.0513	615	31.55
Walking rapidly (5.80 mph)	0.1667	10	1.67
Driving an automobile	0.0438	600	26.28
Attending a movie	0.0206	132	2.72
			279.97

Energy expended in physical activity per week =
279.97 k Cal./kg × 70 kg (body weight) = 19597.9 k Cal. or 2800 k Cal./day.

For calculations of energy expenditure for various activities generally the following Table compiled by Professor Mary S. Rose is used.

Table 8.5. Total Energy Expenditure Per Hour Under Different Conditions of Muscular Activity

From of Activity	*Calories per hour* Per 70 Kilograms (Average Man)	Per Kilogram	Per pound
1	2	3	4
Sleeping	65	0.93	0.43
Awake lying still	77	1.10	0.50
Sitting at rest	100	1.43	0.65
Reading aloud	105	1.50	0.69
Standing relaxed	105	1.50	0.69
Hand sewing	111	1.59	0.72
Standing at attention	115	1.63	0.74
Knitting (23 stitches per minute on sweater)	116	1.66	0.75
Dressing and undressing	118	1.69	0.77
Singing	122	1.74	0.79
Tailoring	135	1.93	0.88
Typewriting rapidly	140	2.00	0.91
Ironing (with five-pound iron)	144	2.06	0.93
Dishwashing (plates, bowls, cups and saucers)	144	2.06	0.93
Sweeping bare floor (38 strokes per minute)	169	2.41	1.09
Bookbinding	170	2.43	1.10
"Light exercise"	170	2.43	1.10

(contd.)

1	2	3	4
Shoemaking	180	2.57	1.17
Walking slowly (2.6 miles per hour)	200	2.86	1.30
Carpentry, metal working, industrial painting	240	3.43	1.56
"Active exercise"	290	4.14	1.88
Walking moderately fast (3.75 miles per hour)	300	4.28	1.95
Walking down stairs	364	5.20	2.36
Stoneworking	400	5.71	2.60
"Severe exercise"	450	6.43	2.92
Sawing wood	480	6.86	3.12
Swimming	500	7.14	3.25
Running (5.3 miles per hour)	570	8.14	3.70
"Very severe exercise"	600	8.57	3.90
Walking very fast (5.3 miles per hour)	650	9.28	4.22
Walking up stairs	1100	15.8	7.18

By the use of these estimates the probable food requirement for a person of 70 kilograms (154 pounds) may be calculated very simply, as, for instance, in the following examples:

8 hours, of sleep at 65 Calories = 520 Calories
2 hours, light exercise at 170 Calories = 340 Calories
8 hours, carpenter work at 240 Calories= 1920 Calories
6 hours, sitting at rest at 100 Calories = 600 Calories
3380 Calories

Textbook of Physiology by Tigerstedt gives estimates of food requirements for different degrees of activity which may be useful in checking results calculated as above:

2000-2400 Calories per day suffice for a shoemaker.
2400-2700 Calories per day suffice for a weaver.
2700-3200 Calories per day suffice for a carpenter or mason.
3200-4100 Calories per day suffice for a farm labourer.
4100-5000 Calories per day suffice for an excavator.
Over 5000 Calories per day are required by a lumberman.

Lusk gives the following summary of energy needs of women at work at typical occupations as investigated by Becker and Hamalainen in Finland:

A seamstress sewing with a needle required 1800 Calories.

Two seamstresses, using a sewing machine, required 1900 and 2100 Calories, respectively.

Two bookbinders required 1900 and 2100 Calories.

Two household servants, employed in such occupations as cleaning windows and floors, scouring, knives, forks and spoons, scouring copper and iron pots, required 2300 to 2900 Calories.

Two washerwomen, the same servants as the last above named, required 2600 and 3400 Calories in the fulfillment of their daily work.

The Use of Tables of Recommended Energy Allowances or Systems for Determining Total Energy Need

In this approach the individuals' caloric needs are estimated by making use of the accepted tables recommended energy allowances. Such tables were prepared. On the motion of its Food and *Nutrition Board,* the (U.S.) *National Research Council* in 1948 revised its *Recommended* (Daily) *Dietary Allowances* for healthy adult maintenance to read, as regards Calories, as follows:

Man (154 lb., 70 kg.)				
Sedentary	2400 Calories a day			
Physically active	3000	"	"	"
With heavy work	4500	"	"	"
Woman (123 lb., 56 kg)				
Sedentary	2000	"	"	"
Moderately active	2400	"	"	"
Very active	3000	"	"	"

Caloric requirements proposed above are used in U.S.A. For international use the Tables of Caloric requirements have been prepared by Food and Agriculture organization of U.N. (FAO).

Table 8.6. The Calorie Requirements of the FAO[1]

Age Group	Males Cal.	Both Sexes Cal.	Females Cal.
0-1		1120	
1-3		1300	
4-6		1700	
7-9		2100	
10-12	2500		2400
13-15	3100		2600
16-19	3600		2400
20-29	3200		2300
30-39	3104		2231
40-49	3008		2162
50-59	2768		1990
60-69	2528		1817
70+	2208		1587

1Based of FAO reference standards of body size and environmental temperature (Adult weights: male 65 kg; female 55 kg. Temperature: 10 ° C.)

In the use of this method the NRC table of daily dietary allowances in used for U.S.A. and the FAO tables are used on international scale. As in factorial method so also in this method there are some limitations for assessing energy need.

The Recommended Allowances for Energy

The daily recommended Caloric allowances proposed by NRC as given in Table 8.6

Table 8.7. The Daily Recommended Calorie Allowances of the NRC

Age, years	Males Cal.	Both Sexes Cal.	Females Cal.
1	2	3	4
Infants, up to 1 yr		kg × 115 ± 15	
1-3		1300	
3-6		1600	
6-9		2100	

1	2	3	4
9-12	2400		2200
12-15	3000		2500
15-18	3400		2300
18-35[1]	2900		2100
35-55[1]	2600		1900
55-75[1]	2200		1600
		add 200 Cal. for 2nd and 3rd trimesters of pregnancy	
		add 1000 Cal. for lactation	

[1]70-kg (154 lb) man and 58-kg (128 lb) woman.

Suitable adjustments are desirable in these for various factors such as for age, stress periods of pregnancy, lactation,growth etc.

The adjustment for Age, Body size etc.

The recommendations in above table are for person of age 18-35 having 58 kg body weight.

The needs for energy decrease with age and so the energy allowances are reduced by 5% per decade during the age 35-55 years by 8% per decade between 55-75 years and by 10% beyond 75 years.

To make adjustments in weights various formulas are used depending upon the age and sex..

For Men

At age 25 (18-35)years

The requirement is [725+31 W] Cal (W= Weight in kg)

At age 45 (35-55) years

It is calculated by using the formula (650+28 W) Cal

At 65 years (55-75) years

The formula used is (559 + 23.5W) Cal.

The Corresponding Formula for women is

At age 25 years (525 + 27 W) Cal.

At age 45 years (475 + 24.5 W) Cal.

At age 65 years (400 + 20.5 W) Cal.

The FAO System

The need for a system of international energy standards was recognized during the World War II. Since that time two reports (3, 4) have been prepared by the Committee on Calorie Requirements of the FAO for assessing the caloric requirements, which with appropriate adjustments can be applied to different people in different parts of the world.

The FAO system derives caloric requirements for adult populations from the measurements of two "reference" persons as does the NRC system. Tables of numerical values are then used to assess energy needs of populations based on variations in body size, age, and environmental temperature. For example, according to the FAO system, the energy allowance for 21-years-old women weighing 55 kg and living in a climate where the annual temperature averages 10°C is 2300 Cal. (Table 8.6). If these same women lived in part of the world where the average temperature was 20 °C rather than 10 °C, their energy requirement would be 5 per cent less or 2185 Cal. At age 64, these same women would have a Caloric allowance 21% less (1817 Cal.) than their needs at age 21.

The FAO energy requirements for childhood and early adolescence are assessed independently of the reference requirements, except as they pertain to environmental temperature. In late adolescence, ages 16 to 20, The caloric requirements are based on body size as well as climate. The additional energy allowance for reproduction and lactation has been assessed as 40,000 extra Cal. per pregnancy and 180.000 extra Cal. per lactation. This modern statement of assessing energy needs is highly tentative and open to testing and further research. However, it has been used satisfactorily in providing for the food production programs in many countries.

Energy Allowances for Pregnancy and Lactation

Although the basal metabolism does not seem to be greatly increased per unit of weight in pregnancy, yet by virtue of her increase in weight the pregnant woman has a larger total energy requirement. The effect of increased weight is likely to be offset to some extent by the decrease in activity. During lactation, when the entire nutritive requirement of the nursing infant is being met through the mother, the energy needs of the latter are greatly increased. Production of milk involves an extra energy requirement beyond the actual energy value of the milk secreted, and the food allowance should provide accordingly. Liberal feeding of the nursing mother is not only important for the conservation of her own bodily resources but may prolong the period of lactation and thus be of great value to the child as well.

The National Research Council recommends allowances of 2500 Calories per day for women in the latter half of pregnancy, and 3000 Calories for women in lactation, stating that these figures "seek a middle ground within the somewhat broad range of present professional opinion."

Total Energy Requirements of Children

The relatively large energy requirement of children as compared with that of adults is due to a higher basal metabolism, vigorous muscular activity, and stimulation from their food intake, which must be liberal to support the storage of protein and fatty or fat-like material in the body for growth.

With children, the energy requirement includes an additional provision for growth. In studies of infants 7 to 9 months old, Rubner and Heubner found a storage of 12% of the energy value of the food consumed, and Camerer found a storage of 15 per cent of the energy and 40% of the protein of the diet. An allowance of 10 to 15% of the calories of the basal metabolism is generally considered a safe allowance for storage except in the periods of most rapid growth.

In order to provide adequately for all contingencies and support the rapid growth which is normal at this age, it is estimated that a vigorous child will require during the greater part of the first year about 100 Calories of food per kilogram of his body weight per day. But in cases of artificial feeding, since the digestive tract must be gradually educated to handle the milk of a different species, it will often be necessary to feed much less than 100 Calories per kilogram per day at first and gradually increase the food allowance, under the advice of the physician.

From the end of the first year until growth is completed the food requirement increases, but not so rapidly as does the body weight, so that while the allowance of food becomes larger per day it becomes smaller per kilogram of body weight.

Effects of Fatness on Langevity of Life

On the basis of various studies conducted by life insurance companies it has been found that the best weight for a given height is that of normal person at the age of 25 years.

Young people were advised to attain this much weight and older people were advised not to allow any increase in their weight beyond this weight at the age of 25 years.

Table 8.8. Pounds of Weight for Height as of Ages 25 And 30

Height	*Women*		*Men*	
	Age 25	*Age 30*	*Age 25*	*Age 30*
4 ft 8 in.	109	112		
4 ft 9 in.	111	114		
4 ft 10 in.	113	116		
4 ft 11 in.	115	118		
5 ft 0 in.	117	120	122	126
5 ft 1 in.	119	122	124	128
5 ft 2 in.	121	124	126	130
5 ft 3 in.	124	127	129	133
5 ft 4 in.	128	131	133	136
5 ft 5 in.	131	134	137	140
5 ft 6 in.	135	138	141	144
5 ft 7 in.	139	142	145	148
5 ft 8 in.	143	146	149	152
5 ft 9 in.	147	150	153	156
5 ft 10 in.	151	154	157	161
5 ft 11 in.	154	157	162	166
6 ft 0 in.	158	161	167	172
6 ft 1 in.			173	178
6 ft 2 in.			179	184
6 ft 3 in.			184	190
6 ft 4 in.			189	196

While the body's weight may sometimes be significantly influenced by its water balance, in the large majority of cases overweight means over-fatness.

And over-fatness almost always means that the intake of food calories has been out of proportion to the expenditure of energy *by the person concerned.*

There are other reasons for a person to be over weight such as inherent tendency to be over weight, functioning of endocrine glands etc.

To control body weight, there is tendency to administer thyroid, thyroxine etc. to increase basal metabolism but it should the avoided. If necessary it should be done under strict medical control.

To increase energy metabolism muscular exercise is useful but strenuous exercises may be dangerous to people who are over weight as well as those who are no longer youth. They should remember the maxim expounded by Dr Mary S. Rose that only form of exercise essential to control of body weight is the exercise of the intelligence.

The reduction in body weight can also be achieved by reducing the intake of Calories. However, one should not proceed two drastically and one should not change his plans even if sudden fluctuation of a few pounds are observed because any weight reduction plan should aim not at spectacular results but at steady moderate progress, it is well when reducing to deduct about 500 Calories from the daily intake which would keep the body weight constant.

9

Mineral Elements in Food and Nutrition

9.1. Introduction

Minerals comprise the ash of biological materials remaining after the organic substances have been completely oxidized. The bulk of the total ash from animal body represents the skeletal minerals. Some minerals present in animal body apparently are contaminants that gain entrance through food, water or air e.g. *barium, nickel, lead* and *tin*. They are present in trace quantities and are not active in cellular metabolism.

The minerals known to be essential and which are present in fairly large quantities are *calcium, phosphorus, potassium, sodium, chloride, magnesium* and *sulfur.* The principal elements present in micro-quantities are *iron, copper, cobalt, manganese, zinc, iodine* and *molybdenum.* Accumulating evidence indicates that *selenium* and *chromium* also function in metabolic systems and that organic *arsenic* compounds promote growth in some species.

Furthermore traces of mineral elements such as aluminum, boron-vanadium and other have been found in animal tissues; but as yet there is no conclusive evidence that any of these has a special biological function.

Mineral elements are present in the body in combination with organic compounds, in combination with other inorganic ions, and as free ions for example, some of the calcium present in blood is bound to protein, some is present as free ions. In bone, phosphorus exists in combination with the mineral calcium. In body cells phosphorus is in organic combination with lipids to form phospholipids, with proteins to form phosphoproteins, and with other compounds to form substances important in the metabolic processes of the body.

9.2. Elementary Composition of the Body

From various estimates it has been concluded that carbohydrates, lipids, and proteins (which are compound containing carbon, hydrogen, oxygen and nitrogen) with water constitute about 96% of body weight. The remainder 4% is made up of mineral elements. Table 9.1 lists these elements as estimated by the data from many sources and Table 9.2 lists these as estimated by Clarke (1920) on the basis of elaborate studies of as much of the earth's solid crust as with in it ten miles of sea level, together with oceans and other waters of the earth's surface and air of its weighable atmosphere.

Table 9.1. Approximate Elementary Composition of the Adult Human Body

(Data from many sources)

Chemical Elements	*Percentage*
1	2
Oxygen	65.
Carbon	18.
Hydrogen	10.
Nitrogen	3.0
Calcium	1.5-2.2
Phosphorus	0.8-1.2
Potassium	0.35
Sulfur	0.25
Sodium	0.15
Chlorine	0.15
Magnesium	0.05
Iron	0.004
Manganese	0.0003
Copper	0.00015
Iodine	0.00004

(Contd.)

1	2
Cobalt	(σ)
Zinc	(σ)
Others found, but of doubtful function	

Table. 9.2. Approximate Elementary Composition of the Earth's Crust with its Oceans and Atmosphere
(Clarke)

Chemical Elements	*Percentage*
Oxygen	50.02
Silicon	25.80
Aluminum	7.30
Iron	4.18
Calcium	3.22
Sodium	2.36
Potassium	2.28
Magnesium	2.08
Hydrogen	0.95
Titanium	0.43
Chlorine	0.20
Carbon	0.18
Phosphorus	0.11
Sulfur	0.11
Fluorine	0.10
Barium	0.08
Manganese	0.08
Nitrogen	0.03
Others in lesser amounts	

The prominence of *oxygen* in the elementary composition of our bodies is, of course, largely due to the fact that about two-thirds of the body weight is water; but also oxygen is a constituent of nearly all of the compounds in the body.

Its prominence as a constituent both of water and of the organic body-stuffs gives *hydrogen* a high place in the quantitatively arranged list of the body's essential elements, and accounts for its constituting a higher percentage of the body than of its environment.

Of *carbon* and also of *nitrogen* the body contains about 100-fold higher concentration than does its environment. This is chiefly due to the fact that the body tissues are so largely compound of carbon and nitrogen compounds.

9.3. Functions of the Minerals

General Functions

The two roles carried out by minerals are

(*i*) as building substances, and

(*ii*) as regulatory substance.

They serve in the following three ways as structural constituents (building substances).

(1) As constituents of the bones and teeth, giving rigidity and relative permanence to the skeletal tissues.

(2) As essential of the organic compounds which are the chief solid constituents of the soft tissues (muscles, blood cells, etc.).

(3) As components in compounds essential to the functioning of the body: iodine is present in thyroxine, zinc in insulin, cobalt in vitamin B_{12}, sulfur in thiamine, iron in hemoglobin, and other compounds in tissue cells.

In regulation of body processes their functions are as follows:

(1) They contribute to the osmotic pressure of body fluids.

(2) They contribute to the maintenance of approximate neutrality in the blood and body tissues by helping to protect against the accumulation of either too much acid or too much base (alkali).

(3) They make possible normal rhythm in the heart beat.

(4) They help to maintain a normal response of nerves to stimuli.

(5) They are essential for blood clot formation.

(6) As soluble salts (electrolytes) held in solution in the fluids of the body, giving these fluids their characteristic influence upon the elasticity and irritability of muscle and nerve, supplying the material for the acidity or alkalinity of the digestive juices and other secretions, and yet maintaining the approximate neutrality of the body's fluids as well as their osmatic pressure and solvent power.

A man under average conditions of diet, activity and health usually excretes daily from 20 to 30 grams of mineral salts, consisting mainly of chlorides, sulfates, and phosphates of sodium, potassium, magnesium, and calcium (as well as variable small amounts of ammonium salts from the protein metabolism).

9.4. Calcium and Phosphorus

Calcium: The human body contains about 22g Ca/kg fat-free body weight. Well over 90% of all body calcium is concentrated in the hard structures of bones and teeth. Though the precise composition and structure of bone salt are not known, it is generally assumed to resemble a hydroxyapatite similar to $Ca_{10}(PO_4)_6(OH)_2$. Traces of other minerals such as magnesium, sodium, and strontium in combination with phosphates and carbonates or citrates are adsorbed on the surface of bone crystals or trapped in lattice-like network characteristic of bone. Some minerals such as strontium are probably incidental contaminants and are not essential to bone structure.

The muscles contain probably more magnesium than calcium. The blood contains more calcium then magnesium and in the blood most of the calcium is in the plasma, while of magnesium the blood cells contain more than plasma.

9.5. Functions of Calcium

Calcium serves two important functions in the body i.e.:

(*i*) The building of bone and teeth, and

(*ii*) The regulation of certain body processes.

Building Bones and Teeth

The need for calcium for building the skeletal structure is, of course, greater during the years of growth, but the need does not cease when full growth is attained. Once bone is formed, it continues to change, with processes of building new bone and destroying old going on simultaneously.

Calcium together with other mineral elements gives rigidity and performance to bones and teeth by virtue of which it is possible for bones to be the support of the body, providing the rigid structure to which muscle tissues is attached. Bone forms protective cavities for vital organs—heart and lungs in the chest cavity, the brain in the cranial cavity. Although bone will withstand almost as much weight as cast iron before breaking, it is itself light in weight.

The various minerals present in bone are deposited in an organic framework of protein known as the organic matrix. Minerals form 60 to 70% of the weight of dry bone, and organic matter 30 to 40% of the dry bone; fresh bone is 15 to 25% water. The protein is generally *collagen*, which is quite insoluble. The combination of minerals and organic matter can be readily demonstrated by placing bone in a weak acid solution (ordinary household vinegar can be used), which dissolves the salts, leaving the flexible organic matter in the shape of the original bone.

Teeth, like bone, contain both inorganic and organic matter, with the inorganic portion forming the major part. *Enamel*, the outermost covering, is about 99.5% inorganic matter; *dentin*, the portion beneath the enamel and surrounding the tooth pulp, about

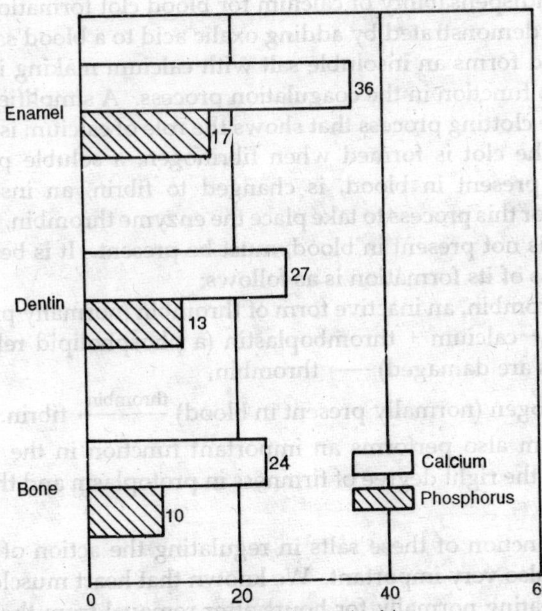

Fig. 9.1. The average calcium and phosphorus content of enamel, dentin, and bone.

77%; and *cementum,* the calcified portion covering the root of the tooth, is about 70% inorganic matter.

Enamel, the hardest tissues in the body, contain 36% calcium and 17% phosphorus, which are more of the minerals than is contained in any other tissue. Dentin is 27% calcium and 13% phosphorus (Fig. 9.1). Although exchange of minerals between enamel and saliva takes place, unlike bone, the enamel of the tooth has no capacity to repair itself after a portion has been injured mechanically or through decay.

The organic matter of teeth is mainly protein. In enamel the protein is a *keratin,* the most insoluble of proteins. In dentin, like bone, the protein is collagen.

Regulatory Functions of Calcium

That the calcium ion is necessary to the coagulation of the blood, has long been known and frequently cited as an example of the great importance of calcium salts to the animal economy.

The indispensability of calcium for blood clot formation, can be clearly demonstrated by adding oxalic acid to a blood sample. Oxalic acid forms an insoluble salt with calcium making it unavailable to function in the coagulation process. A simplified version of the clotting process that shows the role of calcium is given below. The clot is formed when fibrinogen, a soluble protein normally present in blood, is changed to fibrin, an insoluble protein. For this process to take place the enzyme thrombin, which normally is not present in blood, must be present. It is believed the process of its formation is as follows:

Prothrombin, an inactive form of thrombin (normally present in blood) + calcium + thromboplastin (a phospholipid released when cells are damaged) $\longrightarrow$ thrombin.

Fibrinogen (normally present in blood) $\xrightarrow{\text{thrombin}}$ fibrin.

Calcium also performs an important function in the maintenance of the right degree of firmness in protoplasm and the soft tissues.

The function of these salts in regulating the action of heart muscle is also very important. We known that heart muscle may be kept beating normally for hours after removal from the body when supplied, under proper conditions, with an artificial circula tion of blood or lymph or a water solution of blood ash. Howell, Leob, and others have studied the part played by various salts.

The sodium salts take the chief part in the maintenance of normal osmatic pressure and have also a specific influence. Contractility and irritability disappear if they are absent, but when present alone they produce relaxation of the muscle tissues. Calcium salts, also, though occurring in blood in very much smaller quantity, are absolutely necessary to the normal action of the heart muscle; while if present in concentrations above normal, they cause a condition of tonic contraction ("calcium rigor"). There is therefore a balance which must be maintained between calcium on the one hand and sodium (and potassium) on the other. Thus it is found that the alternate contractions and relaxations which constitute the normal heating of the heart are dependent in part upon the presence of sufficient but not excessive concentration of calcium salts, and in part upon the quantitative relationship of calcium to sodium and potassium, in the fluid which bathes the heart muscle. Other active tissues of the body doubtless have analogous requirements as to inorganic salts.

9.6. The Calcium Requirement

Calcium is very unevenly distributed among the staple articles of food, many of which are extremely poor in calcium. Milk contains calcium in abundance and green leaves (except of Goosefoot family) are also good sources.

Upto 1920 it was believed that 0.45g/70kg of body weight per day is the calcium requirement of a normal body and an increase of 50% in it was suggested for use in practical dietetics.

With more data available Leitch in 1937-38 found it to be 0.55g of calcium per day for normal human adults irrespective of their body weight.

NRC recommended in 1941 for provision of 0.8g of calcium per day for normal maintenance of either man or woman regardless of muscular activity. It includes the amount required to meet menstrual losses and to provide a bodily store for use in case of pregnancy and lactation in case of woman.

In 1948, NRC raised the recommended allowance for normal adult maintenance to 1.0g of calcium per day making sufficient provision for individual variations.

However, in some parts of the world people are living normally on considerably less calcium than this Recommended Allowance. But further study makes it appear more probable that the most of the people believed to be living on such low calcium levels are in reality getting significant amounts of calcium from sources which we either do not know about or habitually ignore. It is true that the milk supply which is our main sources of dietary calcium is very scanty in some other parts of the world, notably in the Orient, the Arctic, and among some (by no means all) of the native peoples of Africa. But in every case which has been carefully studied it appears not that such peoples thrive on less calcium, but either that they utilize sources of calcium which we neglect or that, in the course of their lifetimes, they are handicapped by their low calcium intakes. "They may get along on it but they are not as well-off in the long run" as those who get more calcium, is a recent biochemical judgment from the Orient.

In adults there may be a long-continued loss of calcium without the appearance of symptoms because the losses from the blood and soft tissues may be replaced by calcium withdrawn from the bones. Bauer, Aub and Albright (1920) and also Cannon (1939) have explained how, in the organism which has been well supplied with food-calcium, serve as a calcium reserve, readily drawn upon whenever there is, or trends to be, a loss of calcium from the blood and soft tissues.

In general, the well-nourished body so uses its supplies as to keep the calcium content (or, more strictly, the concentration of calcium ions) of the *blood* very nearly constant. This relative constancy of the blood calcium is largely due to the *bone trabeculae.* These are crystals of calcium compound which grow from the inner surface of the ends of the bones, projecting from all directions towards the centre of the cavity, as indicated diagrammatically in Fig.9.2.

The more abundant the supply of calcium received from the food, the greater the development of these bone trabeculae, and viceversa. When this fact was first known it was cited as an instance of *functional hypertrophy* but (at first) received only the mechanical interpretation that the ends of the bones were strengthened by abundant development of these trabeculae, as extra braces strengthen a bridge. Now, however, they are given also a more chemical interpretation which is of very important nutritional significance. As the ends of the bones are quite vascular, they admit free circulation of the blood through them and amongst their trabeculae; and the better the trabeculae are developed the

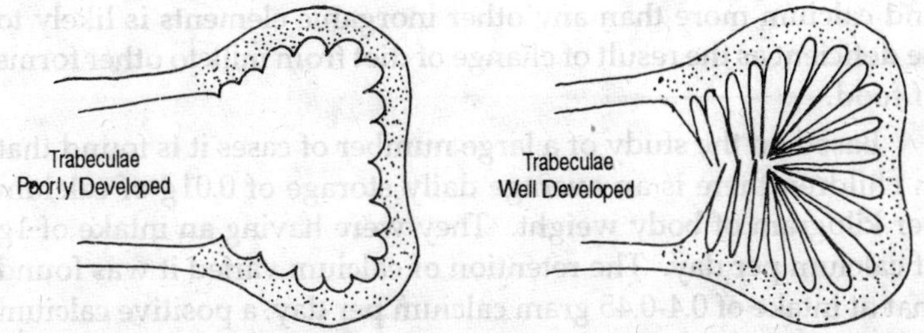

Fig. 9.2. Diagrammatic representations of bone trabeculae showing poor or good development according as the food-calcium intake is low or liberal.

larger is the surface of contact of the blood with this trabecular bone material which "automatically" takes over the storage of any extra calcium which the blood has acquired. And this storing by increased growth of trabeculae both strengthens the ends of the bones and keeps them in good shape (literally) and increases the surface of bone salt from which the blood may promptly replace any loss or expenditure of calcium which may occur incidentally to the widespread functioning of calcium in the body. Thus extra calcium received by the body is not only "passively" stored. It also adds itself promptly and effectively to the body's "working capital" of blood-and tissue-regulatory material.

The diagrammatic representations of Fig.9.2. illustrate extreme cases of the difference between the poor development of these trabeculae in the bone of an animal which has had a diet of low calcium content and the abundant development of the corresponding trabeculae in the bone of an animal which has had a calcium rich diet. This increased means of quick restoration of the calcium concentration of the blood can now be seen as one of the ways in which better diets improve health and longevity.

Calcium Requirements for Pregnancy and Lactation

Pregnant woman need more calcium particularly during the last ten weeks of pregnancy when fetus is storing calcium at a rapid rate. NRC recommended increasing calcium intake unto 1.5g per day during pregnancy and in lactation upto 2.0g per day.

Calcium Requirement of Normal Growth and Development

In children, steady growth with a normally increasing percentage of body calcium require a relatively high calcium intake;

and calcium more than any other inorganic elements is likely to be deficient as the result of change of diet from milk to other forms of food.

Based on the study of a large number of cases it is found that in children there is an average daily storage of 0.01g of calcium per kilogram of body weight. They were having an intake of 1g of calcium per day. The retention of calcium varied it was found that at intake of 0.4-0.45 gram calcium per day, a positive calcium balance is found but at low retention rate and an intake of 0.7 - 0.75g per day gave favourable results of calcium retention. In general we can state that a liberal calcium intake is needed by the body of the infant or child.

The NRC has recommended 1.0g calcium per day upto the age 9 years, 1.2g per day for age 10 -12 years boys and 13 -15 years girls. They recommended 1.0g per day for girls of age 16 -20 years. Boys of age 13 -20 years are recommended 1.4g per day.

Though the present knowledge calls for a much higher estimate of calcium content of properly developed human body than have been taught and for attainment of these higher standards calcium intake should be guite high, but until such time as the numerical estimates of leading investigators have received their final interpretation, the Recommended Allowances of the National Research Council may well be used. In practice these are usually best realized by feeding an average of about a quart of milk per child per day; but this should not be urged too dogmatically for "every" child. An occasional child may have an idiosyncrasy which interferes; but, for general teaching and practice, an average of about a quart of milk per child per day is undoubtedly better than any materially lower average.

9.7. Absorption of Calcium

Factors of Diet Favouring Absorption of Calcium

It has been established that the absorption of calcium is improved if certain nutrients are present in diet. Some such nutrients are vitamin D, protein and ascorbic acid.

Vitamin D: Its presence improves the absorption of calcium specially in those case in which the concentration of available calcium is low in the intestines. Vitamin D improves absorption of calcium when the need of the body for this mineral is comparatively greater as in infancy, pregnancy, lactation, in children with rickets, and adult with osteocalcium. Vitamin D has practically no effect in case of normal adults.

Protein: Poor absorption is observed when diets are deficient in proteins. Increasing the protein content of a low-protein diet improves absorption.

Ascorbic Acid: Though the results of different studies differ but in a particular case on college woman it has been found that the supplementation of diet with additional 25mg of ascorbic acid significantly increased the absorption of calcium.

Factors of Diet Interfering with Calcium Absorption

For calcium to be absorbed it should be in the ionic form and so those conditions which lessen the concentration of calcium ions in the intestine lessen calcium absorption. Two such commonly found substances in diet, that form insoluble calcium salts, are oxalic acid and phytic acid.

Oxalic Acid: It forms insoluble calcium oxalate. It is found in been greens, chard, rhubarb, spinach and cocoa. Thus calcium present in these food items cannot be used however the leafy-green vegetables must be included in diet as they are high in carotene and iron content which are important nutrients indiet.

Though we make use of cocoa liberally with milk in beverages but it has adverse effect on calcium absorption.

Phytic Acid: It occurs in other bran layers of whole wheat, It has been formed that if the diet is adequate in calcium, phytic acid will not have a detrimental effect.

Storage of Calcium: When sufficient quantity of calcium is supplied to the body, calcium may be stored in needle like deposits called *trabeculae* in the end of the bones. When calcium is needed in the tissues or blood, these labile stores in the bones are drawn upon.

As the intake of calcium is lowered, the efficiency of the body to absorb and retain it increases whereas raising the intake may result in reduced absorption. In the adult the rejection of calcium by the intestine constitutes the chief means of adaptation; the same is true for the young. However, another adaptive mechanism available to the young, but not to adults, is deposition of calcium in the growing bone.

Excretion of Calcium: The body organ through which calcium is excreted are the intestines, the kidney and the skin.

On calcium intake of 1g, the mean daily fecal excretion is about 622mg, urine excretion is 235 mg and dermal excretion is 149 mg though this amount increase in case of profuse sweating.

If the intake of calcium is increased then the amount of fecal excretion increases but there is no effect an urinary excretion. Moreover urinary calcium excretion seems to be independent of blood calcium.

Blood Calcium

Normally the quantity of Calcium in blood is 9-11.5 mg per 100 ml. 50 -60 % of blood calcium is in the form of calcium ions and the remaining is bound to protein.

Parathormone (a hormone of parathyroid gland) functions by moving calcium from bone to blood. Vitamin D mediates the movement of labile calcium from bone, under conditions of need for the mineral, to maintain the content of blood at a normal level.

Deficiency of Calcium

Insufficient calcium in diet limits growth in the young. In a deficiency state the concentration of calcium serum decreases to low levels. Tetany, the diagnostic clinical symptom of calcium deficiency, is associated with *rickets,* and osteomalacia which occur at advanced stage of deficiency, osteoporosis is one of the most common disorders of bone and one associated with aging. The bone tissue is normal in composition but reduced in amount. Resorption a normal process in bone, proceeds at a greater rate than dues bone formation in osteoporosis.

In addition to a low calcium intake, the lack of certain hormones (estrogens and androgens) and vitamin D are recognized as factors related to osteoporosis. In the treatment, therefore, it is recommended that not only dietary supplements of calcium be used but also the hormones and vitamin D be explored as curative agents.

9.8. Food Sources of Calcium

In our diet milk and milk products are the major sources of calcium. Other important sources is leafy green vegetables. Broccoli is a good source, citrus fruits and legumes are fair sources, meat, grains and nuts provide the least calcium.

Calcium values of some typical food are listed in Table 9.3.

Table 9.3. Calcium Values of Some typical Foods

Food	*Measure*	*Calcium, mg*
Milk	1 c, 8 oz	288
Cheese, American Cheddar	1 oz	212
Mustard greens	1/2 c	97
Ice cream	1/8 qt	87
Kale	1/2 c	74
Oranges	1 med	67
Broccoli	1/2 c	66
Cottage cheese, creamed	1/4 c	53
Lime beans	1/2 c	38
Green beans	1/2 c	31
Egg	1 med	27
Bread, whole wheat	1 sl	23
Peas	1/2 c	19
Peanut butter	2 tbsp	18
Bread, white enriched	1 sl	16
Cream, light	1 tbsp	16
Oatmeal	1/2 c	11
Potato	1 med	9

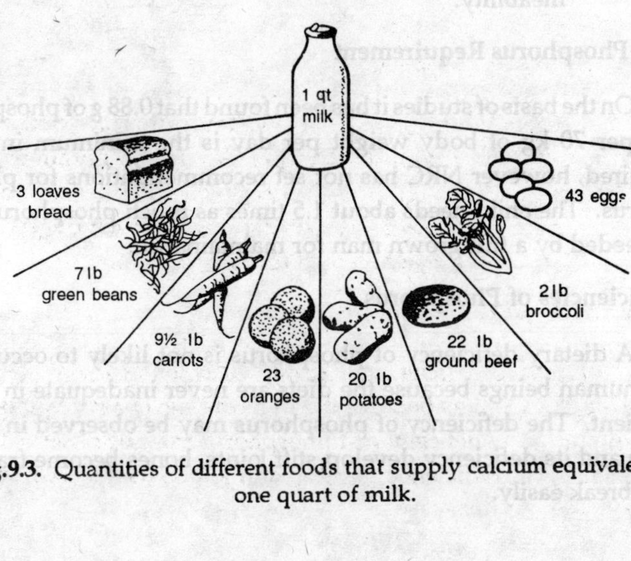

Fig.9.3. Quantities of different foods that supply calcium equivalent to one quart of milk.

9.9. Phosphorus

It is an important constituent in every body tissue and constitutes about 1% of body weight. In body it is only next to calcium. It occurs in bones and teeth in combined form along with calcium. It occurs in fluids and soft tissues as a constituent of many compounds which are essential in active metabolism. It is widely distributed in food.

Functions of phosphorus: Some of important functions are:-

(*i*) It helps in growth and development of the skeleton and its maintenance.

(*ii*) It plays an important role in metabolic processes of all cells.

(*iii*) It helps in the utilization of many nutrients that enter the body.

(*iv*) Phosphorus is a constituent of the high energy compound ATP and so is necessary for energy transductions essential for all cellular activity. The oxidation of carbohydrate leading to the formation of ATP also requires phosphorus since phosphorylation is essential step in metabolism.

(*v*) Phospholipids are constituents of all cellular membranes and are active determinants of cellular permeability.

The Phosphorus Requirement

On the basis of studies it has been found that 0.88 g of phosphorus per 70 kg of body weight per day is the minimum intake required, however NRC has not set recommendations for phosphorus. The child needs about 1.5 times as much phosphorus as in needed by a full grown man for maintainance.

Deficiencies of Phosphorus

A dietary deficiency of phosphorus is not likely to occur in the human beings because the diets are never inadequate in this nutrient. The deficiency of phosphorus may be observed in animals and its deficiency develop stiff joints, bones become fragile and break easily.

Food Sources of Phosphorus

It is widely distributed in both plant and animal foods. Protein-rich foods like meat, poultry, fish, and eggs are good sources of phosphorus, are abundant in supply, and are well-liked foods in the United States. Cereal grains provide phosphorus in good amount, whole grain more than the highly-milled product. The

Table 9.4. Phosphorus Values of Some Typical Foods

Food	*Measure*	*Phosphorus, mg*
Liver, beef, fried	2 sl, 3" × $2\frac{1}{4}$ × 3/8"	311
Milk	1 c, 8 oz	234
Haddock, fried	3 oz	211
Pork chop, Ioin, fried	3 oz	200
Beef, round, cooked	3 oz	195
Lamb, chop, fried	3 oz	185
Cheese, American Cheddar	1 oz,1" cube	139
Baked beans, no pork	1/2c	110
Cottage cheese	1/4c	106
Oatmeal	2/3c	105
Egg	1 med	101
Shredded wheat	1 c	93
Ice cream	1/8qt	78
Broccoli	2/3c	76
Lima beans	1/2 c	62
Bread, whole wheat	1 sl	60
Corn	1/2 c	43
Orange	1 med	35
Grapefruit	1/2 med	32
Bread, white	1 sl	21

higher phosphorus content of the whole-grain products, however, may be misleading because of the greater content of phytin phosphorus which is not readily utilized by the body. Dried beans and eggs contain appreciable amounts of phosphorus, milk and dairy products are excellent sources. Vegetables and fruits, as a whole, are a rather low in phosphorus content (Table 9..4).

9.10. Iodine

It is now fully established that the normal functioning of thyroid gland depends on the adequate supply of iodine in the body. A deficiency of iodine through a few generations may lead to retardation in physical development as also in mental development.

Though the amount of iodine in the body is infinitesimally small (about 20-30 mg), most of it is concentrated in the *thyroid gland.*

In the body it occurs in the bound form as bound to organic compounds.

Iodine and the Thyroid Gland

The thyroid gland is located at the base of the neck. It consists of two lobes, one on either side of the trachea, connected by an isthmus across the front of the trachea. Normally the gland weighs 20 to 25 gm. An insufficient intake of iodine may result in an enlargement of the gland.

The thyroid is one of several endocrine glands. They are sometimes designed as *glands of internal secretion,* or *ductless glands.* Each produces one or more secretion which it pours directly into the blood stream. The secretions of the endocrine glands are known as hormones, a term derived from the Greek meaning to *excite* or *arouse.* They are chemical substances, each with a particular function within the body. The hormones influence growth, nutritional processes, and other specific physiological activities. Thyroxine is the main hormone secreted by the thyroid gland.

It is now a well established fact that iodine is intimately connected within the activity of thyroid gland. The characteristic physiological effects of administration of thyroid gland appear to be directly proportional to the iodine content of the gland administered. The thyroid gland secretes a substance *thyroxine* and the inadequacy of thyroid secretion leads to diseases such as *goiter, cretinism, myxedema.* The thyroid utilizes simple iodide in the preparation of thyroxine perhaps directly and perhaps in part through intermediate substances. Normally the small quantity of iodide contained in food and drink furnishes sufficient iodine both for proper functioning of thyroid gland and the production by it of the hormone needed to regulate metabolism through out the body. In case of inadequate supply of iodine the thyroid gland gets enlarged and it cause goiter (an iodine deficiency disease).

Seaweeds and sea water have long been the familiar sources of iodine. In regions where the people live largely upon sea food, and the atmosphere and drinking water are constantly receiving the iodine-containing salt spray blown in from the sea, the intake of iodine is presumably adequate and in such regions goiter is very rare; but in regions too remote or too mountainous to receive significant amounts either directly or indirectly from the sea, goiter is much more common. Woman and girls are afflicted with endemic goiter more commonly than men and boys.

The WHO Study-Group on Endemic Goiter recommended that "...all food salts should be iodized compulsorily in any country or area in which goiter is endemic, local variations in incidence of disease being disregarded".

On occasion, rumors circulate that the use of iodized salt is harmful to health because of the iodine content. The World Health Organization Study Group on Endemic Goiter states this: "In no country in which iodine prophylaxis has been used on a community scale, has this measures had any adverse effects on the health of the population." From the report of The Third Conference on Nutrition Problems in Latin America, this statement concerning the prophylactic use of iodine explains further that "... all reports of unfavourable effects which have been investigated have proved to be false or explainable on the basis of coincidence."

Iodine Content and Requirement of the Body

Evidently the body has a more or less definite nutritive requirement for iodine. Qualitatively this requirement might be stated as a sufficient amount of iodine to meet the daily losses from the body and maintain such store as is needed to provide for the manufacture and the distribution throughout the body of sufficient amounts of thyroxine (thyroid hormone) to support a normal rate of physiological activity.

According to Marine, if the iodine content of the thyroid is maintained above 0.1 per cent *of its solid matter,* goiter does not develop. According to the estimates of Kendall and Plummer a full grown healthy adult has about 15 mg of iodine in thyroid gland and the rest (10 mg) in the rest of the body. Most of the iodine in the body is chiefly in the form of thyroxine, which has been distributed by the thyroid and is serving to control metabolism in all the active tissues of the body.

Fellenberg estimated that the normal human adult requires about 0.000014 gram of iodine daily and that, when larger amounts are furnished by the food and drink, an easily mobilized reserve store of iodine is built up in the body.

Though still there is no consensus, among the experts, about the amount of iodine required in normal nutrition.

The Food and Nutrition Board of the National Research Council (NRC) estimates that a desirable daily intake of iodine is 0.002 to 0.004 mg per kilogram of body weight or a total of 0.15 to 0.30 mg for the adult. They state that "this need is met by the regular use of iodized salts; its use is especially important in *adolescence* and *pregnancy*."

The prevention of goiter in regions whose soils and waters are very poor in iodine is a nutritional problem whose immediate solution may depend not so much upon detailed knowledge of iodine contents of foods as upon the use of methods which lie largely in the province of the health officer.

The above-noted success of Marine and Kimball in preventing the development of goiter through the giving to the school child of a little iodide in drinking water, naturally suggested the addition of iodide to public water supplies, and this has been done in several communities.

Two other methods have also received favourable attention: the administration of iodine compounds in chocolate tablets or some equivalent palatable form, and the addition of a small proportion of sodium iodide to table salt intended for household use.

Turrentine of the United States Department of Agriculture has emphasized the possibility that it may prove advantageous to give iodine in a form less readily soluble and less rapidly absorbed into the circulation than is a simple iodide solution, and has advocated the use of kelp and particularly preparation of the species *Macrocytis pyrifera* which he finds to be particularly rich in iodine; and Adolph and Whang (1932) find the *Laminaria religiosum* of the Chinese seacoast to be also a rich sources of iodine.

There seems now to be no reasonable doubt that iodized salt can be made a satisfactory means of supplying the nutritional need for iodine.

Recommended Allowances for Iodine

The National Research Council has recommended an intake of iodine of 100 to 150 mg daily for the adult. The need may be greater for the adolescent and pregnant or lactating woman.

Iodine Content of Foods

Though a general view is that the ordinary food contain no iodine (except sea foods) yet the analysis of a variety of foods carried out by McClendon shows the presence of iodine in trace amounts in all of them soil and fertilizer conditions. Vaught and London determined the iodine content of whole meals and individual foods served on metabolic diets and on regular house diets at the Clinical Center, National Institute of Health. The metabolic diet contained from 15 to 219 mg and the regular house diets from 65 to 529 mg per day. The iodine content of food composites in each of seven food categories as determined by Vought and London is presented in Table 9.5. The authors stated that because of the skewed distribution, the median is a better centering constant than the mean.

Marine or deep-sea fish and shell fish are high in iodine content. The anadromous group of fish (those fish that spend a part of the time in sea water and a part in fresh), to which salmon and sea trout belong, contain more iodine than the fish that remain all the time in fresh water but less than most of the fish that remain at sea. The leaves and flowers of plants (spinach, turnip greens, and broccoli) appear to have higher iodine concentration than the roots.

A supplement to the iodine intake in goitrous regions becomes essential. Iodized salt is an effective means of providing the supplement. The amount of iodine added to salt in the United States is 0.01 per cent and is in the form of potassium iodide. It is not compulsory by law that iodine be added to salt, but it is voluntarily

Table 9.5. Iodine Content of Composites of Food Categories

Food Category	*No. of Samples*	*Iodine (mg/wet kg) Mean ± S.E.*	*Median*
Sea foods	7	660 ± 180	540
Vegetables	13	320 ± 100	280
Meat products	12	260 ± 70	175
Eggs	11	260 ± 80	145
Dairy products	18	130 ± 10	139
Bread and cereal	18	100 ± 20	105
Fruits	18	40 ± 20	18

added by the manufactures. A nationwide survey revealed that 20% of the families never use iodized salt, 4% use it a part of the time, and 76% use it exclusively. Vought and London reported that the median amount of salt added at the table by their subjects was 1.59 gm per day. If this were iodized salt, an estimated 122 mg of iodine per day would be added to the diet.

In Table 9.6 some more data about the amount of iodine present in various food stuffs is indicated.

Table 9.6. Iodine in Foods from Goitrous and Non-goitrous Regions: parts Per Billion of Dry Matter

Kind Of Food	*Goitrous Regions*	*Non-goitrous Regions*	*Authority*
1	2	3	4
Wheat	1-6	4-9	McClendon
Oats	10	23-175	McClendon
Carrots	2	170	McClendon
Carrots	—	507	Okla. Agr. Expt. Sta.
Lettuce	—	618	Okla. Agr. Expt. Sta.
Potatoes	85	226	McClendon
Cabbage	—	776	Adolph and Whang
Cranberries	—	26-35	Morse
Asparagus	—	946	Okla. Agr. Expt. Sta.
Radishes	—	994	Okla. Agr. Expt. Sta.
Tomatoes	—	379	Okla. Agr. Expt. Sta.
Milk	265-322	572	Remington and Supplee
Butter	140	—	McClendon

1	2	3	4
Sea foods:			
Codfish	—	5,350	U.S.Bureau of Fisheries
Conch	—	1,140	U.S.Bureau of Fisheries
Crabmeat	—	1,460	U.S.Bureau of Fisheries
Flounder	—	1,480	U.S.Bureau of Fisheries
Oysters	—	1,800-3,500	U.S.Bureau of Fisheries
Red Snapper	—	1,440	U.S.Bureau of Fisheries
Salmon	—	570-2,200	U.S.Bureau of Fisheries
Shrimp	—	1,100	U.S.Bureau of Fisheries
Cod liver oil	—	7,670	U.S.Bureau of Fisheries
Cod liver oil	—	3,000-13,000	Holmes and Remington

Functions of Iodine

The iodine is an essential component of *thyroxine* and so the physiological functions of thyroxine are those of iodine also.

The thyroxine molecule consists of four atoms of iodine and it resemble closely the amino acid tyrosine as shown below:

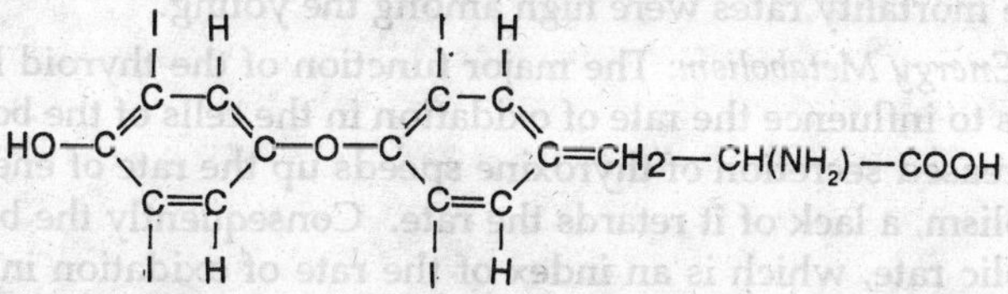

Thyroxine was first isolated from the thyroid gland by Kendall at the Mayo Foundation, Rochester, Minnesota, in 1915. Not until eleven years later was it produced synthetically. Harington and Bager of England accomplished the feat.

Some of its functions are as follows:

In Growth and Development: Thyroxine is necessary for the normal growth and development of the young of all species. In case of under-section the growth may be retarded, and if the reduction is severe and prolonged it may result in failure to mature both physically and mentally.

Children suffering from a severe deficiency of the thyroid secretion are cretins. Their growth is retarded and their development arrested; their facial features appear coarse and swollen; the skin is thick, dry, and pasty in appearance, and often deeply wrinkled. The tongue is enlarged, the lips are thickened and usually stay ajar.

Cretinism generally occurs in those parts of the world where iodine shortage exists.

One of the symptoms of thyroid deficiency in the adult is myxedema. The skin and subcutaneous tissues, particularly of the face and extremities, are thickened and puffy. The face is characteristically expressionless, the person lethargic and inactive.

In pregnancy and Lactation: Iodine is essential for normal reproduction in both man and animal. It has been observed that women frequently develop a goiter during pregnancy, indicating a greater need for the thyroid hormone.

Observations on animals provide evidence of the need for it for reproduction. A prolonged and severe lack may results in sterility, or if young are born they may be deformed. Farms animals in low-iodine regions showed abnormalities in reproduction that are now prevented by providing a sufficient amount of the mineral. Pigs were born without hair; sheep, swine, horses, and cattle developed enlarged thyroid glands during pregnancy, and the mortality rates were high among the young.

In Energy Metabolism: The major function of the thyroid hormone is to influence the rate of oxidation in the cells of the body. An increased secretion of thyroxine speeds up the rate of energy metabolism, a lack of it retards the rate. Consequently the basal metabolic rate, which is an index of the rate of oxidation in the cells, is also an indicator of the normality of thyroid function. An elevated basal rate is indicative of hypersecretion of the hormone, a low rate indicates hyposecretion.

The other laboratory procedures use to assess the state of thyroid functions are (*a*) determination of protein-bound iodine (PBI) in blood serum, and (*b*) observations on the utilization of radioactive iodine. The protein-bound iodine is mostly thyroxine. It is found to be low in hypothyroidism and elevated in hyperthyroidism.

Using radioactive iodine makes it possible to trace the utilization of an iodine dosage in the body; iodine normally present is not radioactive. An observation commonly made is the uptake of iodine by the thyroid gland. In general the hyperfunctioning gland takes up more iodine than the normal; the hypofunctioning gland takes up less.

Metabolism of Iodine

Absorption: Iodine is readily absorbed both in organic and inorganic forms. Within 3 to 6 minutes after the administration of radioactive iodine to fasting individuals, it has been detected in the hand using the Geiger-Muller counter to measure the speed of absorption take a capsule of (0.2 gm) potassium iodide and swallow it and in a few minutes the saliva gives a blue colour with starch paste, indicating the presence of iodine.

Most of the iodine is absorbed from the small intestine. Some, however, enters the blood stream directly from the stomach. It can even be absorbed from the skin but not to any degree of practical importance.

Utilization: After absorption into the blood, the iodine is taken up by the thyroid gland and other tissues. The thyroid gland concentrates the element and serves as a storehouse for it. In man the ratio of iodine in the thyroid to that in the blood is about 25 to 1.

After the iodine is concentrated in the thyroid gland it is formed into these iodine-containing compounds: monoiodotyrosine, diiodotyrosine, thyroxine, diiodothyronine, and triiodothyronine. These compounds are present in the gland in a complex known as thyroglobulin. Of various Iodine compounds, thyroxine is the main. It leaves the gland to enter the blood stream and carries on the functions of the hormone through out the body.

The body is conservation of its iodine supply. When thyroxine breaks down, some of the iodine is saved for reuse. The salvaged iodine joins that absorbed from the gastrointestinal tract in a common pool for use.

Excretion: The chief pathway of excretion of iodine is by way of the kidney, with lesser amounts through the intestine, and in perspiration. During lactation some is secreted into the milk. During the laying season some of the iodine fed to hens is recovered in the eggs.

Marine considers (1935) that the substance actually secreted by the thyroid is probably iodothyroglobulin (commonly called thyroglobulin) but that thyroxine seems to be the active part of the thyroglobulin molecule, natural and synthetic thyroxine both having essentially the same effect as natural thyroid secretion, and showing the maximum degree of the effect somewhat more quickly.

Marine suggests that the exact way in which thyroxine increases oxidative processes in the cells may perhaps be not yet fully known; but that there is considerable evidence that epinephrine (adrenine, adrenaline) and thyroxine may work together in this process. There are also reasons for believing that thyroxine is always present and acting, though in differing degrees according to the amount secreted by the gland, where as the throwing of epinephrine into the circulation by the adrenal glands may be essentially an emergency response. In this case, the two would act together in times of markedly accelerated oxidation rate, while thyroxine alone may suffice to maintain oxidation at such rates as obtain in times of relative quiescence.

Antithyroid Compounds

The term antithyroid compounds is used for a number of substances that inhibit the formation of the thyroid hormone.

Drugs: One group of drugs functions by inhibiting the uptake of iodine by the thyroid gland. Thiocyanate is such a drug. However, if the level of iodine in the blood is sufficiently high, iodine may enter the thyroid, presumably by diffusion. A second group of drugs exerts its effect on the functioning of the thyroid gland a step beyond the process of iodine concentration. These compounds appear to block thyroxine synthesis even though the supply of the iodide ion is adequate. Such drugs include thiourea, thiouracil, phenol derivatives, and cobaltous chloride.

Antithyroid Compound in Foods: There appears to be little doubt but that there are factors in some foods that increase the need for dietary iodine and these are called "goitrogenic" as they increase susceptibility to goiter caused due to iodine deficiency. It is believed that these substances may be partly responsible, for the simple goiters that appear in both man and animal at times, in spite of an intake of iodine that would normally be considered adequate.

The discovery that goitrogenic factors exist came from experimental studies with animals. It was in 1928 at Johns Hopkins University that rabbits fed almost exclusively on fresh cabbage were observed to develop enlarged thyroid glands. It was a fortuitous finding, for the investigators were actually seeking information on a certain disease condition unrelated to goiter.

Since the early study with cabbage, an antithyroid compound has been identified in the seeds of most of the mustard family and the edible portion of some plants (cabbage, kale and rape). The substance is known as goitrin and has been established as (-)-5-vinyl-2-oxazolidinethione. A precursor of goitrin, progoitrin, is present also in the seeds of some plants and has thus far been identified only in the edible portion of rutabagas and white turnips.

Progoitrin is active only when it gets converted to goitrin. It was first believed that the enzyme that converts progoitrin to goitrin was present in the food but could be destroyed by heat. It is now known that progoitrin can be converted to goitrin by enzymes in the intestine. Thus cooked food as well as raw containing the compounds are potentially goitrogenic.

It may be that continuous ingestion of small amounts of goitrin or other unidentified goitrogens that may exist, may change normal thyroid hormone synthesis. The effect would be expected to be more severe if only the minimal quantity of iodine required by the body were supplied in the diet.

9.11. Iron

Iron is essential to the process of oxidation in the body. It is a constituent in compounds which are necessary for the transport of oxygen to the cells and for oxidation in the cells.

The human body contains 75 mg Iron/kg fat free body weight i.e. in adults its amount in 3-5 g. Most of the iron occurs as protein chelates in which hence compounds predominate. The hence molecule is comprised of ferrous or ferric iron in the centre of a porphyrin ring. *Hemoglobin* contains four porphyrin units bound to protein globin. *Myoglobin*, a compound like hemoglobin, found in skeletal and heart muscles, contains only one ferrous porphyrin group per molecule. Though bother these (i.e. hacmoglobin and myoglobin) enter into a reversible combination with oxygen, myoglobin has the greater affinity and due to this property it serves as a cell reservoir of oxygen. About 75% of the total body iron is contained in these two compounds.

Iron is also present in erythrocytes of blood, and in serum in ferric form bound to a specific β-globulin, transferrin (siderophilin). The quantitative ability of transferrin to buid iron is known as *iron-binding capacity* of serum. Practically no ionic iron exists in the animal body.

About 26% of the total body content of iron is stored in cells of liver, spleen and bone as *ferritin* and *hemosiderin*.

Functions of Iron in Body

Some of the important functions of iron are as follows :

(1) It is an essential elements of the chromatin substances which in some sense preside over the most vital activities of the cells.

(2) It is also an essential element of the hemoglobin which is the outstanding substance of the red cells (erythrocytes) of the blood, and thus of the blood's property of taking up oxygen in the lungs and carrying it to all the tissues in which oxidation occurs.

(3) Iron likewise is an essential element of the myoglobulin (muscle hemoglobin) which is closely related, chemically and functionally, to hemoglobin, acting with it to regulate oxidation-reduction (redox) systems.

(4) Both iron and copper participate further in tissue oxidation reductions through the catalytic actions of cytochromes and cytochrome oxidises which have been estimated by Schultze (1947) to "mediate about 90% of the energy transfer associated with the aerobic phase of tissues respiration."

(5) And finally, iron is an essential part of other highly important body enzymes.

In addition to these five active forms of iron, the body may also carry a reserve in the form of ferritin, a non-diffusible substance from which iron can be liberated as needed for hemoglobin formation.

Copper is in some way involved in the process of hemoglobin formation. While its action is catalytic in the sense that it does not appear as a constituent of the hemoglobin formed yet this action of copper in hemoglobin formation and regeneration is now regarded as part of the normal nutritional process. Hence copper is now counted among the nutritionally essential; elements; and the study of iron and copper in nutrition, of the nutritional anemias and hemoglobin formation and regeneration, are so closely interdependent as to be scientifically inseparable.

The primary role of iron in animals can be over simplified as influencing oxidation. Actually hence compounds serve as carriers of oxygen to tissue cells and transporters of hydrogen to molecular oxygen as a part of the cellular electron transport system. In iron deficiency, the lowered capacity to provide oxygen is largely responsible for the fatigue and apathy characteristic of iron deficiency anemia. This type of anemia occurs exclusively in women and young children. This is by far the most common form of anemia due to nutritional deficiency of iron.

Soon after its absorption iron is incorporated into hemoglobin. This process takes place in the bone marrow where new red cells are formed. Experimental evidence shows that within 4 hours the iron (*i*) travels to bone marrow (*ii*) gets incorporated into the hemoglobin portion of new red blood cells and (*iii*) returns to circulation.

The life span of erythrocytes is about 120 days and about 20,000 billion erythrocytes are there in our body, so they get destroyed at the rate of 115 million per minute.

In lungs oxygen combine with hemoglobin to form *oxyhaemoglobin* that carries oxygen to the tissues and releases it there. *Hemoglobin* from which oxygen has been released is called *reduced hemoglobin* which then returns to the lungs by way of various circulation and cycle is repeated.

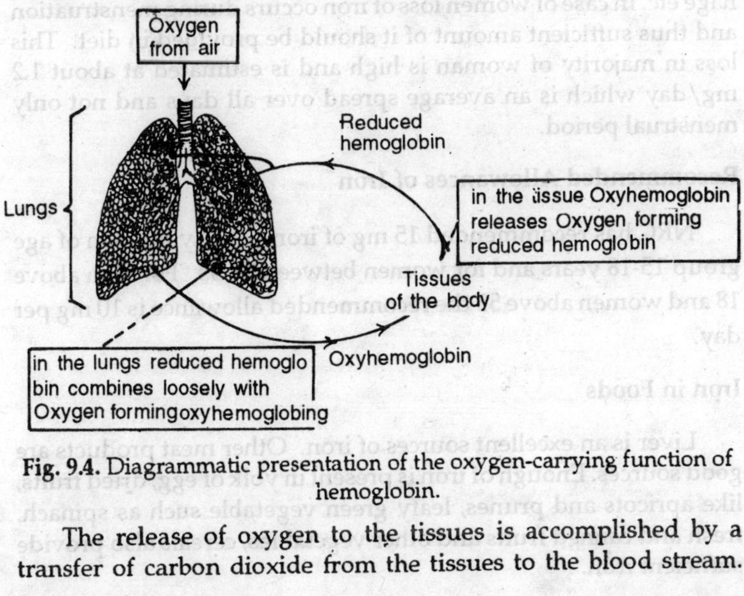

Fig. 9.4. Diagrammatic presentation of the oxygen-carrying function of hemoglobin.

The release of oxygen to the tissues is accomplished by a transfer of carbon dioxide from the tissues to the blood stream.

About 10% of the carbon dioxide is carried by the hemoglobin; the major portion, however, is carried as bicarbonate ion.

There is a small quantity of iron in blood plasma where it comes from: (*i*) absorbed from the gastrointestinal tract, (*ii*) break down of hemoglobin, and (*iii*) released from stores in the body.

The level of iron in plasma is considered a sensitive index of the state of iron metabolism in the body.

In muscles iron is present as (*i*) myoglobin, and (*ii*) as a constituent of certain enzymes.

The iron containing enzymes in muscles make possible the oxidation of carbohydrate, fat and protein with in the intact cell. These enzymes are *cytochromes, catalase, peroxidases* etc.

Excretion of Iron

Only very little iron is excreted. The amount of iron that is extracted from the blood stream into the intestine in case of normal adult is 0.02 to 0.05 mg per day. Only about 0.2 mg per day is excreted in urine.

Significant quantities of iron are lost by body during loss of blood which may be due to blood donation, abnormal hemorrhage etc. In case of women loss of iron occurs during menstruation and thus sufficient amount of it should be provided in diet. This loss in majority of woman is high and is estimated at about 1.2 mg/day which is an average spread over all days and not only menstrual period.

Recommended Allowances of Iron

NRC has recommended 15 mg of iron per day for men of age group 15-18 years and for women between 18-55. For men above 18 and women above 55 the recommended allowance is 10 mg per day.

Iron in Foods

Liver is an excellent sources of iron. Other meat products are good sources. Enough of iron is present in yolk of egg, dried fruits, like apricots and prunes, leafy green vegetable such as spinach, fresh and canned fruits and other vegetables, cereals also provide sufficient iron.

Molasses is rich in iron content. If a mixed diet of cereals, milk, meat, vegetables and fruits we taken the required amount of iron is provided to the body. The iron content of some food item is given in Table 9.7.

Table 9.7. Iron Values of Some Typical Foods

Food	*Measure*	*Iron, mg*
1	2	3
Cereal products		
Rice, white, cooked, enriched	1/2 c	0.7
Bread, white enriched	1 sl	0.5
Bread, whole wheat	1 sl	0.6
Dairy products		
Cheese, Cheddar	1 cu in.	0.2
Milk, whole	1 c	0.1
Egg	1 med	1.1
Fish		
Salmon, cooked	3 oz	0.7
Fruit, fresh		
Orange	1 med	0.5
Apricot	3	0.5
Apple, pear	1 med	0.4
Fruit, dried		
Raisins	1/2 c	2.8
Apricot	1/2 c	2.5
Prunes, cooked	8-9 sm	2.2
Legumes		
Red kidney beans, canned	1/2 c	2.3
Meat		
Beef liver, cooked	2 oz	5.0
Beef, pork, cooked	3 oz	2.6
Chicken, cooked	3 oz	1.4
Nuts		
Peanut butter	1 tbsp	0.3
Molasses		
Blackstrap	1 tbsp	3.2

Contd.

1	2	3
Light	1 tbsp	0.9
Vegetables		
Spinach, cooked	1/2 c	2.0
Peas, cooked	1/2 c	1.5
Potato, cooked	1 med	0.7
Tomato, raw and cooked	1 sm, 1/2 c	0.7
Broccoli, cooked	1/2 c	0.6
Carrots, cooked	1/2 c	0..5
Head lettuce, cabbage, raw	1 c	0.5

Absorption of Iron

Absorption of iron: Iron is absorbed directly into the blood stream. The process may occur in all parts of the intestinal tract with the exception of the colon; absorption from that area is not definitely established. The duodenum is the location of greatest absorption, with the amount progressively decreasing from jejunum to ileum.

In man iron is much more efficiently absorbed in the ferrous (reduced) state than in the ferric (oxidized) form. The iron in food, however, is predominantly in the ferric form. Reducing substances present in foods are thought to change some of the ferric iron present to the ferrous form. Basics of this assumption is the finding that ascorbic acid, a reducing substance, when fed with ferric iron enhances absorption but has no effect on the absorption of ferrous iron.

Iron movement through the intestinal cell is unidirectional; that is, absorption from the intestine into the blood takes place, but re-excretion does not occur from the blood back into intestine.

The finding that some mechanism exists for the control of iron absorption was established through the use of radioactive elements. An ingenious study was done by Moore and his associates at Washington University. Persons with iron-deficiency anemia absorbed as much as 45 to 64% at the same level of intake. Values in general for iron absorption suggested by Moore and Dubach are, for normal persons, 5 to 10% (Fig. 9.4) and for iron-deficient persons 10 to 20% of the iron in the food consumed. Individuals with a greater need for iron absorb a greater amount.

A relationship between iron absorption and the rate of erythrocyte formation has been observed. It has been found that at the higher altitude absorption and red cell formation increased markedly over the values observed at sea level. By the end of a month at the higher altitude, however, the rates of absorption and cell formation returned to the sea-level values; adaptation had occurred.

At present the mode of regulation of iron absorption is not understood. Absorption is of particular importance for iron because the capacity for elimination by the normal pathways, the kidney and re-excretion into the intestine, is negligible. Thus any control of the amount in the body must be at the time of absorption.

For the past quarter century the theory has been held that the ferritin content of the intestinal mucosa controlled the absorption of iron. More recent studies have not supported this theory.

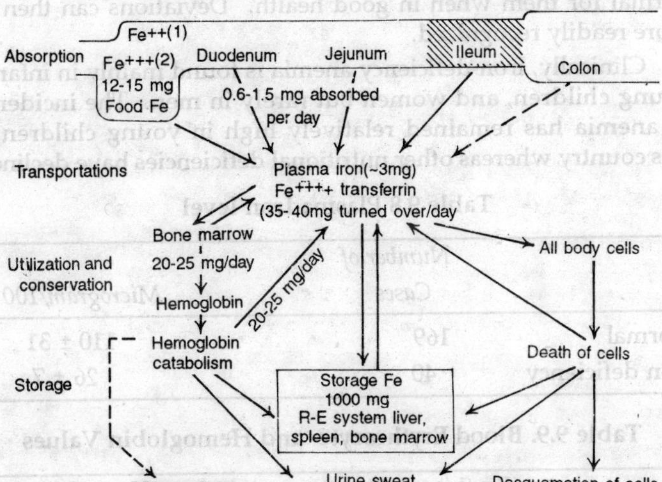

Fig. 9.5. Diagrammatic outline of iron metabolism in adults. (1) Fe + + - ferrous ion. Fe + + + - ferric ion.

Diseases Due to Deficiency of Iron

The two common forms of iron deficiency are: (*i*) latent iron deficiency, and (*ii*) Manifest iron deficiency.

In *Latent iron deficiency* the available iron stores get depleted, plasma iron level get reduced, and the iron binding capacity of the blood is increased. It means that more of transferrin (a protein that takes an iron) is free and uncombined.

In *Manifest iron deficiency* the person appears weak, hallid and has frequent head aches. The hemoglobin level is lower than normal and the RBC's are smaller than normal. This results in lower oxygen carrying capacity and anemia.

The iron and hemoglobin content of the blood in iron-deficiency anemia is markedly reduced. As shown in Table 9.8, the plasma iron level may be reduced to one-fourth that of normal. With hemoglobin although the level is found to vary widely among apparently healthy individuals, values 25% or more below normal are generally considered to indicate a condition of anemia. For men the normal range is from 14.0 to 18.0 gm per 100 ml; for women it is lower, varying from 11.5 to 16.0 gm per 100 ml (Table 9.9). It is wise for persons to know the level of hemoglobin that is normal for them when in good health. Deviations can then be more readily recognized.

Clinically, iron-deficiency anemia is found mainly in infants, young children, and women but rarely in men. The incidence of anemia has remained relatively high in young children of this country whereas other nutritional deficiencies have declined.

Table 9.8 Plasma Iron level

	Number of Cases	*Microgram/100 ml*
Normal	169	110 ± 31
Iron deficiency	40	26 ± 7

Table 9.9. Blood Erythrocyte and Hemoglobin Values

	Erythrocyte Count, millions/cu mm		*Hemoglobin, gm/100 ml*	
Age	*Mean*	*Range*	*Mean*	*Range*
End 6th month	4.6	3.9-5.3	12.3	10.0-15.0
End 12th month	4.6	4.0-5.5	11.6	9.0-14.6
End 4th year	4.7	3.8-5.4	12.6	9.6-15.5
End 8th year	4.7	3.8-5.4	12.9	10.3-15.5
End 12th year	4.8	3.8-5.4	13.4	11.0-16.5
14 years and over				
Males	5.4	4.6-6.2	15.8	14.0-18.0
Females	4.8	4.6-5.4	13.9	11.5-16.0

In infants the prevalence of anemia may be because of two factors: the low iron stores in the newborn caused by low intakes of iron during pregnancy and the use of cow's milk formulas without sufficient supplementation of iron-containing foods. In women the condition may be due to large menstrual losses or the increased needs of pregnancy. In men, unless there is some abnormal blood loss, microcytic hypochromic anemia seldom, if ever, develops. On a global level a major cause of iron-deficiency anemia is hookworm infestation with the attendant blood loss. The parasites attach themselves to the mucosa of the small intestine and draw blood from the submucosal blood vessels.

Blood donors experience a lowering of the hemoglobin level with each donation. The decrease may average 2.3 gm per 100 ml of blood with the removal of approximately 1 pint (555 ml), as found in a study of 200 persons at the University of Iowa. The mean hemoglobin level prior to the donation for this group was 12.8 gm. The length of time required for hemoglobin to return to the predonation level varies with individuals. It may be as short as 2 to 3 weeks for some or as long as 3 to 4 months for others. The average time required by the 200 Iowa persons was 50 days. For women the period of recovery is longer than for men. The difference among individuals is explained on the basis of variability in iron stores.

The administration of medicinal iron and the adherence to certain dietary precautions hasten the restoration of the hemoglobin level after giving blood. Medicinal iron administered as 1 gm of iron and ammonium citrate per day shortened the period from an average of 50 to 35 days after the first donation, with progressively less effect after subsequent donations.

Increasing the protein content of the diet was found to hasten the restoration of hemoglobin in a study of University of Nebraska college women. Diets containing 50, 75, and 90 gm of protein daily were fed to 129 young women who were contributors to the local blood bank. Only those who received 90 gm of protein daily had hemoglobin values of the predonation level in six week's time.

10

Vitamins

10.1. Introduction

A new era in nutrition was ushered in with the discovery of vitamins. It was one in which small things in the diet assumed great importance. The percentage of body weight attributable to vitamins is very minute. Nevertheless, the amount, even though small, is indispensable for normal functioning.

Vitamins are chemically unrelated organic compounds that are grouped together because each is essential and is required for specific metabolic reactions with in the cell.

Jean Dumas (1800-1884) was the earliest man of science to question the adequacy of a diet composed of only proteins, carbohydrates, fat and salts. This observation of Dumas was not based on any experimental scientific facts but on the observations on citizens of France. When the France was under the siege of Germans (1870-71)food was scarce. There was no milk for children. Artificial milk was prepared from proteins, fats, carbohydrates and salts. This combination was however found to be disastrous to the young. It was from this observation that Dumas concluded that there was something lacking in combination of then known nutrients essential for life.

The organic compounds other than carbohydrates proteins, and fats that are necessary to maintain normal health, growth and nutrition are called *vitamins.*

It may be noted that vitamins are not used in building cells or as energy source but they act as catalysts in biological processes, their deficiency causes serious diseases.

The vitamins are complex organic molecules, however for sake of simplicity they are represented by letters such as A,B,C,D,E,K.

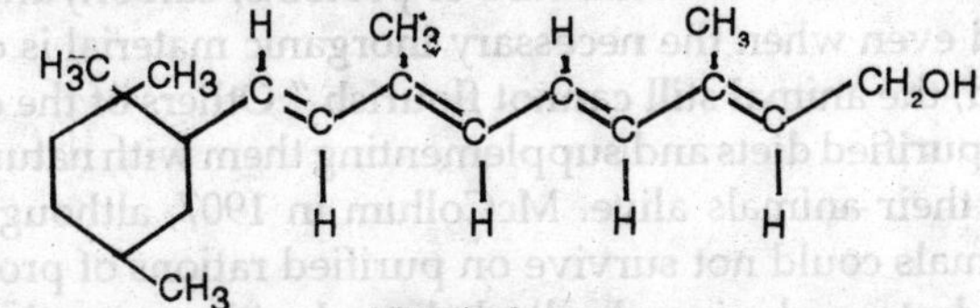

Vitamin A

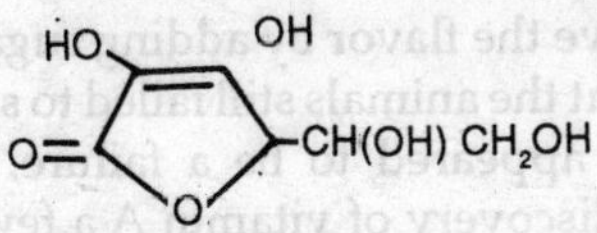

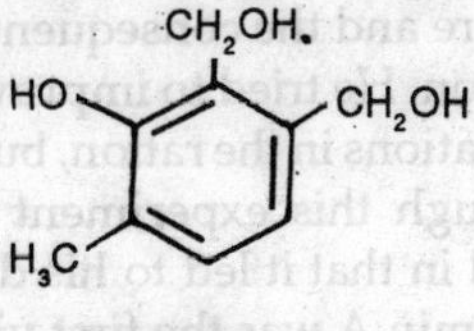

Vitamin C

Vitamin B6

10.2. Discovery of Vitamins

Significantly, the vitamins were discovered not by their presence in the diet but because of their absence. Early evidence of the existence of vitamins came from the search for treatments of certain human diseases that persistently plagued the people. The two diseases to name were *scurvy* and *Beri-beri.*

In 1747 relief from *scurvy* was enjoyed by a few of the British Navy. The sailors were served lemons and oranges and a remarkable recovery from scurvy was observed.

The persons in Japan Navy were suffering from *Beri-beri.* They ate only white rice. However, when vegetables, meat and fish were added to their diet (in 1884) the incidence of beri-beri decreased.

It was about 150 years after these observations it was only in the early 1900's that scurvy and beri-beri were accepted as diseases caused due to deficiency in diet.

As the deficiencies in diet could be responsible for disease was a new concept so it was adopted with reluctance.

Animal experiments that led to the discovery of vitamins included those of Pekelharing in 1905 at the University of Utrecht, who made the important observation that a diet of casein, egg albumen, rice flour, lard, and salts kept his mice alive only four weeks. When he added milk to the mixture the mice remained healthy.

Sir Frederick Hopkins of England was the most advanced thinker of his time on animal nutrition. He said in 1906 that ".... no animal can live on a mixture of proteins, carbohydrates, and fats, and even when the necessary inorganic material is carefully supplied, the animal still cannot flourish." Others of the era were feeding purified diets and supplementing them with natural foods to keep their animals alive. McCollum in 1907, although aware that animals could not survive on purified rations of protein, fat, carbohydrate, and mineral salts, believed with many others of his time that the failure to survive was due to the unpalatability of the mixture and the consequent refusal to eat a sufficient amount of the ration. He tried to improve the flavor by adding sugars and other variations in the ration, but the animals still failed to survive. Even though this experiment appeared to be a failure, it was successful in that it led to his discovery of vitamin A a few years later. Vitamin A was the first vitamin to be discovered and it was called fat soluble vitamin A.

There seemed to be only one factor needed to supplement the purified diet at the time of the discovery of vitamin A. In a couple of years, however, it was recognized that not one, but two factors were lacking in the purified diet for normal growth, one soluble in fat, the other soluble in water. Later of course, numerous new fat-soluble and many additional water-soluble factors were identified. Each is discussed in the chapters that follow. A chronological summary of the isolation and syntheses of the various vitamins follows (2).

Year	*Isolation or Identification*	*Synthesis or structure*
1	2	3
1925	Vitamin D by irradiation	
1926	Vitamin B_1	
1928	Inositol	
1931	Vitamin A	
1932	Vitamin C	
1933	Riboflavin	Vitamin C
	Pantothenate	
1935	Biotin	Riboflavin
1936	Anti-egg-white factor	Vitamin D
	Vitamin E	Thiamine
1937		Vitamin A
		α-tocopherol

(contd.)

1	2	3
1938	Nicotinic acid identified as pellagra-preventing Pyridoxine	*dl* α-tocopheral
1939	Vitamin K	Vitiman K Pyridoxine
1940	P-Aminobenzoic acid	Pantothenate
1942		Biotin structure
1945	Folic acid	Folic acid
1948	Vitamin B_{12}	Folionic acid
1955-56		Vitamin B_{12} structure

The term "vitamin" was coined by the polish biochemist, Funk in 1911. It is derived by combining *vita* (meaning essential to life) and *amine* (indicating the chemical structure). However, in 1919 the final "e" was dropped and the word "vitamin" was retained.

Since body cannot synthesize these (except vitamin D) vitamins so they must be provided in diet vitamin D is synthesized in the body. On exposure to ultra violet rays the body develops it (vitamin D) from its precursor present in the skin. Vitamins are regulatory substances, each performing a specific function. They are carried in blood stream to all parts of the body.

10.3. Vitamin A

Vitamin A was the first of the accessory food factors to be identified as a component of specific foods. It is a fat soluble substance and a lack of it was shown to result in necrosis of the cornea is rats that is a condition very similar to an eye disease (xerophthalmia) seen in humans. Mori (1922) established that it is caused due to deficiency of vitamin A in diet. Wald in 1935 discovered that the pigment *rhodopsin* (visual purple), responsible for sight in dim light, contained vitamin A in combination with protein. It has been indicated by varies experiments performed on rats that vitamin A was associated with plants containing the yellow carotene pigments. Moore (1930) demonstrated that the carotenes were related structurally to vitamin A and were converted in *vivo* to the vitamin.

Vitamin A was isolated in large quantities from fish liver oils by Karrer (1931). However, it was only in 1940's that this vitamin was available on commercial scale.

Properties of Vitamin A

Vitamin A is an organic compound found only in animal kingdom. Two forms of vitamin A have been identified; vitamin A_1, which occurs in livers of salt-water fish, and vitamin A_2found in livers of fresh-water fish.

Several isomers of vitamin exist in nature. The former designation of vitamin A_1 and vitamin A_2 and Neo-vitamins A_a and so forth are no longer used; retinal, retinal and retinoic acid are accepted chemical nomenclature (IUPAC, 1960).

(Retinol) vitamin A is pale yellow substance consisting of carbon, hydrogen and oxygen. It is soluble in fat, not soluble in water, stable to heat (upto ordinary cooking temperatures) and destroyed by both oxidation and ultraviolat irradiation. The basis for most chemical determinations for vitamin A is Carr- Price reaction, in which the vitamin forms a blue colour with antimony Trichloride on chloroform.

Vitamin A activity in plants resides in the carotenoid pigments which are precursors to the vitamin in the animal body and are therefore designated the provitamins A. The carteniod pigments are composed only of carbon and hydrogen. The crystals of cartenoid pigments are deep red in colour but in solution intensely yellow. β-carotene is more efficiently converted to vitamin A than α or γ-carotene or cryptoxanthin the β-carotene molecule gives rise to two molecules of retinol (vitamin A) since the carotenoid is in fact, a double retinol structure. Biologically the activity of β-carotene is only about half that of retinol. The β-ionone ring is essential for vitamin A activity.

Vitamin A is measured in International units (IU). The IU is equal to 0.3 μg of vitamin A alcohol. Equal biological activity is afforded by 0.6 μg of pro-vitamin β-carotene.

In America its activity is expressed in USP which is the same as IU.

Functions of Vitamin A

Growth: Better growth is associated with higher vitamin potency in food. Animals maintained on a vitamin-A-free diet will cease growing when the body is depleted of its vitamin stores. If vitamin A supply is inadequate then the bony structure will suffer growth failure which sometimes may lead to paralysis. Many a times its deficiency leads to blindness.

Epithelial Tissues: Deficiency of vitamin A causes an abnormal condition of epithelial tissues. The specialized functions of the tissues are suppressed and it is transformed to a keratinized (dry, horny) type of epithelium. Its deficiency results in *xeropthalmia* (an eye disease). The disease rarely occurs in USA but is quite common in China, India etc.

Biochemical function: In its only well defined role the vitamin is a constituent of the visual pigment rhodopsin present in the *rod cells* of retina of most, but not all, vertebrates. Iodopsin, the other light sensitive pigment is present in the *cone cells., rods* and *cones* are two types of receptor cells present in retina rods function in dim light and the cones function in bright light and colour vision.

The visual cycle of rhodopsin and iodopsin are believed to be similar; the cycle for rhodopsin (visual purple) is shown in Fig.10.2. In bright light rhodopsin changes to retinene plus protein with a possible loss of some vitamin A. To resynthesize rhodopsin, vitamin A must be reoxidized to retinene and combined with a special protein opsin (Fig. 10.1). If sufficient vitamin A is not available, night blindness may occur. Night blindness is characterized by inability to see in dim light (nyctalopia) and the necessity of a prolonged time to adjust to dim light after exposure to bright light.

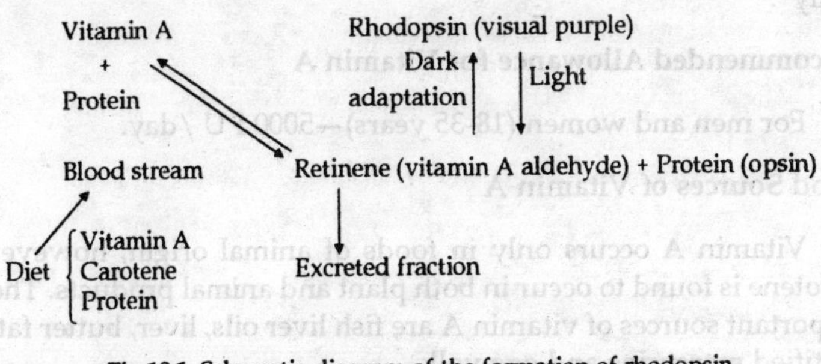

Fig.10.1. Schematic diagram of the formation of rhodopsin.

Absorption

Vitamin A and carotene are absorbed from the small intestines into the lymph system in about 3-5 hours, vitamin A is absorbed more rapidly than carotene. Bile is essential for absorption of carotene. If mineral oil is taken with food and since vitamin A and carotene are soluble in it. Since the oil is not absorbed some of vitamin A and carotene are eliminated with it.

In human body most of the vitamin A is stored in liver and only a small amount in lungs,body fats and kidneys. A normal liver may contain 600,000 I U of vitamin A , enough to supply vitamin needs for one year.

Like other fat soluble vitamins it is excreted by any of intestines. Most of the fat soluble vitamins are excreted by fecal path way and water soluble vitamins by the urinary path way.

Hypecritaninosis A

It is a disease caused due to excessive intake of vitamin A. It is characterized by swelling of feet and ankles, fatigue, lassitude, weight loss and intermittent pains in the shoulders, wrists, knees. Arctic travellers who have consumed polar bear liver, which is extremely high in vitamin A content have manifested symptoms of this disease.

Acute toxicity may occur as an end stage of prolonged chronic toxicity resulting from overdosege over a time period. According to a report of the Council on Foods and Nutrition of the American Medical Association, "there is a definite possibility of harm from prolonged ingestion of vitamin A in excess of 50,000 USP units daily".

Recommended Allowance for Vitamin A

For men and women (18-35 years)—5000 I U /day.

Food Sources of Vitamin A

Vitamin A occurs only in foods of animal origin, however carotene is found to occur in both plant and animal products. The important sources of vitamin A are fish liver oils, liver, butter fat, fortified margarine and egg yolk.

The most important sources of provitamin (caroteue) are the yellow, yellowish red and green vegetables and fruits. e.g. carrots, sweet potatoes, apricots, spinach, tomatoes and kale. Small quantities of vitamin A are also present in nuts, grains, vegetable oils, muscle meats and light coloured fruit and vegetables.

Table 10.1 lists the vitamin A values of some common foods.

Table 10.1 Vitamin A Value of Some Typical Foods

Food	Protion	IU/Portion
Liver, beef, fried	2 oz	30,280
Potatoes, sweet, baked	1 med	8,910
Carrots, cooked	1/2 c	7,610
Spinach, cooked	1/2 c	7,290
Kale, cooked	1/2 c	4,070
Mustard greens, cooked	1/2 c	4,060
Apricots, canned	4 med hf	2,120
Broccoli, cooked	1/2 c	1,875
Peaches, raw	1 med	1,320
Eggs, whole	1 med	590
Ice cream, plain	1/8 qt	370
Milk, whole	1 c	350
Cheese, process	1 oz	350
Orange juice, fresh	1/2 c	245
Butter (average)	1 pat	230
Margarine, fortified	1 pat	230
Bananas	1 med	190
Apples, raw	1 med	50
Pecans	1 tbsp	10
Bread, whole wheat	1 sl	trace
Oatmeal	1/2 c	0

During cooking there is no loss of vitamin A or carotene. Also no loss of these food components occurs during canning and freezing. However, a considerable loss occurs during drying and dehydration.

Any development of rancidity in fats results in destruction of both vitamin A and carotene.

The daily requirements of vitamin A can be met by supply the following meals (Table 10.2):

Table 10.2. Foods Providing the Day's Recommended Allowance of Vitamin A (18-35 Years Age)

Food	*Portion*	*Vitamin A Value, IU*
Liver, beef, fried	2 oz	30,280
Spinach, cooked	1/2 c	7.290
Broccoli, cooked	2/3 c	2.500
Eggs, whole	2 med	1,180
Peach, raw	1 med	1,320
	Total	5,000
Apricots, canned	4 med hf	2,130
Milk, whole	1 pt	700
Beans, green	3/4 c	510
Egg, whole	1 med	590
Butter	1 tbsp	460
Ice cream, plain	1/8 qt	370
Orange juice, fresh	1/2 c	245
	Total	5,005

10.4. Vitamin D

It has been said facetiously that civilization changed vitamin D from a hormone into a vitamin. Certainly the beneficial effect of sunlight in the prevention of rickets was recognized long before there was any indication that vitamins existed. Palm an English physicist, as early as 1890 observed that when sun shine was abundant, rickets were rare. A few years later the concept developed that like beri-beri and scruvy, rickets might be a dietary deficiency disease.

In mid 1920's Steenbock (1924) showed that irradiation of foods produced antirachitic activity. Later the phenomenon was shown to be due to activation of sterols in foods.

In 1921 Mellanky in England produced rickets in puppies by using a mixture of natural foods and then cured it be using cod liver oil. Since by that time cod liver oil was known to contain only vitamin A, so the cure was attributed to vitamin A. Later it was found that even after vatamin A content of food was destroyed by oxidation, the antiricketic potency still remained. The factor responsible for prevention of rickets was named vitamin D and was clearly distinguished from vitamin A also present in oils.

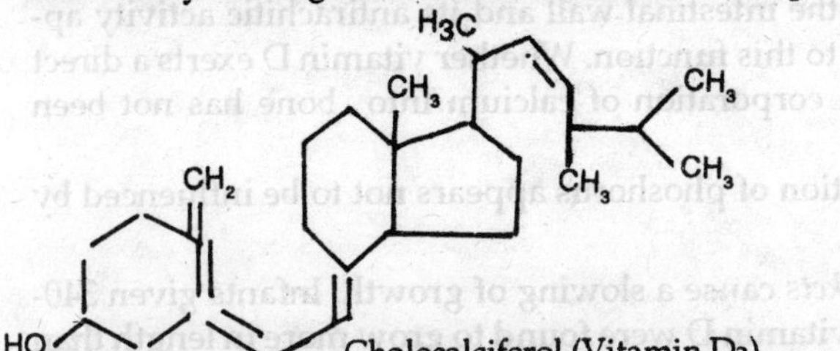

Cholecalciferol (Vitamin D_3)

Vitamin D_3 is formed in human skin on irradiation of 7 - dehydrocholesterol. The irradiation of ergosterol, a pro-vitamin D in plant foods, produces a different substance, designated as vitamin D_2.

The two provitamins of vitamin D are 7 - dehydreocholesterol and ergosterol. The former is present in higher animals and invertebrates where as ergosterol is present in plant kingdom in yeast and certain moulds.

It is a fat soluble vitamin and is soluble in ether, alcohol, chlorofrom, actone etc. It is resistant to heat, oxidation, acids and alkalies.

Vitamin D potency is expressed in International Units (IU). The amount of antiricketic activity brought about by 0.025 ug of the International standard pure crystalline vitamin D_3 is an International Unit (adopted by WHO in 1949) USP is the same as IU.

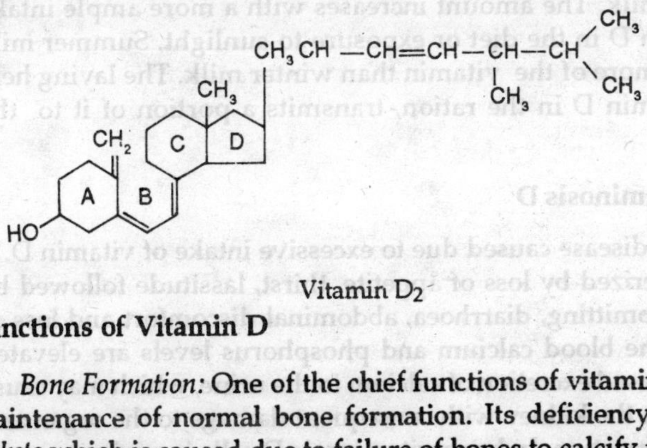

Vitamin D_2

Functions of Vitamin D

Bone Formation: One of the chief functions of vitamin D is the maintenance of normal bone formation. Its deficiency leads to *rickets* which is caused due to failure of bones to calcify normally.

The fundamental role of vitamin D is unknown. Neither a coenzyine function nor a specific work of action has been identified. Vitamin D is known, however, to facilitate the transport of calcium across the intestinal wall and its antirachitic activity appears to be due to this function. Whether vitamin D exerts a direct influence on in corporation of calcium into bone has not been resolved.

The absorption of phoshorus appears not to be influenced by vitamin D.

Growth: Rickets cause a slowing of growth. Infants given 340-400 IU daily of vitamin D were found to grow more in length than those receiving 60 - 135 IU. Giving more than 600 IU did not increase the growth rate further and increasing the vitamin D intake beyond 1800 IU daily decreased growth.

Metabolism of Vitamin D

Vitamin D can be provided to the body through various food sources or concentrates and by activation of the provitamin, 7 -dehydocholesterol, in the Skin. The vitamin taken by mouth is absorbed from the small intestine mainly by way of the lymph system. The process is facilitated by the presence of fat. Bile is essential for normal absorption of the vitamin from the intestaine. The main site of storage of vitamin is the liver with smaller quantities stored in the skin, brain, lungs, spleen and bones. Excretion of vitamin D is by way of the bowel, with no excretion through the kidney.

During lactation there is some transmission of vitamin D into the milk. The amount increases with a more ample intake of vitamin D in the diet or exposure to sunlight. Summer milk contains more of the vitamin than winter milk. The laying hen, with vitamin D in the ration, transmits a portion of it to the egg yolk.

Hypervitaminosis D

It is a disease caused due to excessive intake of vitamin D. It is characterized by loss of appetite, thirst, lassitude followed by nausea, Vomitting, diarrhoea, abdominal discomfort and loss of weight. The blood calcium and phosphorus levels are elevated with increased excretion of calcium in the urine, which may cause deposits in the kidney with consequent damage to the organ and impaired function. In hypervitaminosis D cells in various organs of the body, as well as the arteries and arterioles, become susceptible to abnormal deposition of calcium. Severe intoxication with widespread calcification of soft tissues ultimately may prove fatal it massive dosages are continued.

The recommended allowances of vitamin D is 400 IU daily for children and adolescents.

Sources of Vitamin D

The best sources of vitamin D are fish oils, milk, butter, egg-yolk etc. Vitamin D content of some food sources is listed in Table 10.3.

Table 10.3. Vitamin D Content of Selected Sources

Source	*Measure*	*Vitamin D, IU*
Oil, swordfish liver[1]	1 gm	10,000
Oil, halibut liver[1]	1 gm	1,200
Oil, cod liver[1]	1 gm	100
Milk, whole[2]	8 oz	100
Liver, chicken[2]	2 oz	40
Liver, beef[2]	2 oz	38
Egg yolk[2]	1 med	27
Butter[2]	1 tbsp	4
Oil, corn[2]	1 tbsp	0

Vitamin D present in food is stable in ordinary cooking, heat processing treatments and storage.

10.5. Vitamin E (Tocopherols)

The vitamin E group has been known as *antisterility* vitamin. It was discovered in 1922 by Evans and Bishop; as the fat soluble factor that prevented resorption of fetuses in pregnant female rats and testicular regeneration in males. The name *tocopherol* was derived from the Greek *Tokos* (child birth) and *phero* (to bear), but the influence of tocopherol is vastly greater than the original designation implies.

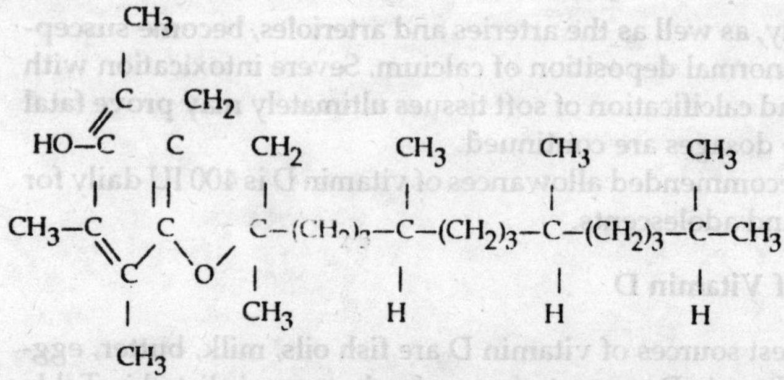

Fig. 10.2. Alpha-tocopherof. (vitamin E).

Several substances designated collectively as tocopherols comprise the vitamin E group. They are all derivatives of 6 - hydrox chroman and contain a 13- carbon isoprenoid side chain.

T ie tocopherols are antioxidants and help in protecting other nutrie its such as vitamin A and polyunsturated fatty acids from destructive oxidation. The biological activity of tocopherlos varies with α- being the most potent.

Vitamin E occurs as a yellow viscous oil. It is a fat soluble vitamin. It is quite stable to acids and heat (in the absence of oxygen). It gets readily destroyed by ultra-violet light, alkalies and oxygen.

Functions of Vitamin E

It acts possibly as an activator in certain enzymatic reactions. It plays an important role in the protection of vitamin A, carotene, ascorbic acid from oxidation in digestive tract and in body cells.

Deficiency of *tocopherols* causes creatiminia and muscular dystrophy in rabbit and rat, encephalomalavia and muscular dystrophy in chicks.

Presently we have no conclusive evidence to show that vitamin E is essential to man. It seems to have no effect an sterility in man. However, studies have shown that those persons who received smallest amounts of vitamin E showed the greatest degree of red cell hemolysis.

The recommended allowances of vitamin E varies between 10- 30 mg daily for adults. Since vitamin E is widely distributed in food so its deficiency is not likely to occur in human beings. An average daily diet has been found to curtain 14 mg of vitamin E.

Food Sources of Vitamin E

The richest sources of vitamin F are found in vegetable oils (such as wheat germ oil, cotton-seed oil), leafy green plants, vegetables, whole grain cereals. Liver, heart, kidney, milk and eggs are the best animal sources.

10.6. Vitamin K (Naphthoquinones)

Vitamin K was identified in 1935 by Dam as a factor present in green leaves which prevented a hemmorhagic syndrome observed in chicks maintained at a low fat diet. The new fat-soluble vitamin was named vitamin K from the Danish Word *koagulation.*

Vitamin K represented a group of substances related to the synthetic compound 2-Methyl-1, 4 - naphthoquinoane (menakione, vitamin K_3. Two forms of vitamin K are found in nature; K_1 occurs in green leaves and K_2 is produced by bacterid synthesis. These, K_1 (phylloguinone) and K_2 (farnoqiunoone) are stable to heat, unstable to alkalig, strong acids, oxidation and light. The synthetic compound, menadione (vitamin K_3 is about twice as active biologically as the naturally occurring vitamins.

Natural compounds are fat soluble but menadione (synthetic compound) is soluble in boiling water.

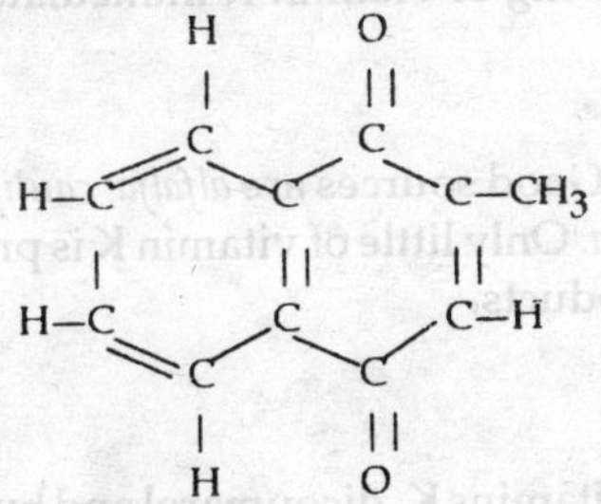

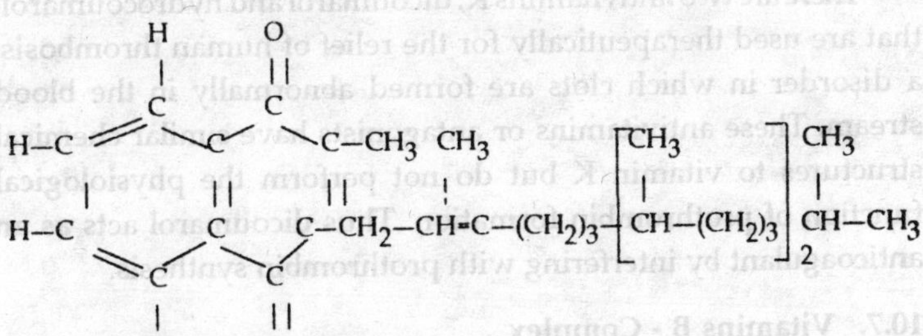

Menadione (Vitamin K_3)

Functions of Vitamin K

It is essential for synthesis of prothrombin, in liver cells, a precursor of thrombin, one of the factors needed for normal blood coagulation.

A deficiency of vitamin K leads to increasing clotting time.

In man the deficiency of vitamin K is seldom caused due to lack of nutrient but caused due lack a faulty absorption of the vitamin or liver disorders that interfere with the synthesis of prothrombin Sometimes the large amounts of sulpha drugs or other antibiotics may destroy the micro - organisms which synthesize the vitamin and the supply then may become low.

It is fat soluble vitamin and so bile is essential for its absorption.

The Food and Nutrition Board states, "with the exception of new born infants, the average diet plus synthesis by intestinal bacteria provide adquate amounts of vitamin K".

It has recommended that vitamin K may be administered to the normal newborn infant, routinely, but is especially indicated for infants with increased susceptibility to neonatal hemorrhage (prematurity, anoxia).... A single parenteral dose of 0.5-1.0 mg or an oral dose of 1.0-2.0 mg is considered adequate for prophylaxis...Infants born to mothers receiving anticoagulant therapy should be given 2.0-4.0 mg of vitamin K immediately after birth.

Sources of Vitamin K

It occurs in plants. Good sources are *alfalfa, cauliflower, cabbage, spinach, kale* and *soybean*. Only little of vitamin K is present in fruits, cereals and animal products.

Antivitamins K

There are two antivitamins K, dicoumarol and hydrocoumarol, that are used therapeutically for the relief of human thrombosis, a disorder in which clots are formed abnormally in the blood stream. These antivitamins or antagonists have similar chemical structures to vitamin K but do not perform the physiological function of prothrombin formation. Thus dicoumarol acts as an anticoagulant by interfering with prothrombin synthesis.

10.7. Vitamins B - Complex

These include thiamine, riboflavin and niacin. This group of B- complex vitamins is important for the will being of every single cell in the body. They are essential for the normal metabolism of food. Their deficiency produces visible characteristic symptoms in both animals and men.

Thiamine (Vitamin B_1)

Beri-beri was known several centuries before its dietary origin was recognized. *Beri-beri* is a nervous disease caused by lack of thiamine in diet. Takkai (1882) demonstrated that the disease *Beri-beri* can be controlled by adding meat and whole grains to diet. It was isolated in 1926 and was synthesized in 1936.

The crystals of vitamin B_1 are colourless having a yeast like smell. They have a salty taste and are soluble in water. It is quite stable in acid solutions but in neutral or slightly alkaline solutions get easily destroyed by heat. Commercially it is sold in the form of thiamine hydrochloride.

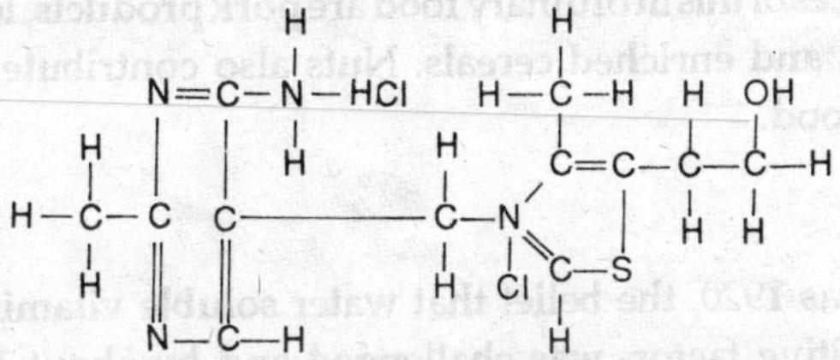

Fig. 10.3. Crystalline thiamine hydrochloride and its chemical formula.

Functions of Thiamine

The longest known functions of thiamine are the *promotion of growth and the prevention of polyneuritis.*

Thiamine promotes the recovery appetite in a more prompt specific way and its deficiency causes characteristically more abrupt loss of appetite. So we can say that it *promotes appetite.*

It is often called the *morale* vitamin because of its ability to restore a healthy mental state in man.

Thiamine functions very importantly in the intermediary metablism presumably acting mainly in the form of its pyrophosphate (cocarboxylase), catalyzes the transformation of pyruire acid and thus helps in carbohydrate metabloism. It has also been found to be concerned in nutritional support of successful pregnancy and lactation.

The recommended allowances for thiamine are 0.5 mg per 1000 cal (1958) but revised in 1963 to 0.4 mg per 1000 cal. Thus for an average adult its requirement is 1.2 mg per day (for females its is 0.8 mg / day).

Either *the microgram (mcg.)* or *the miligram per 100 grams of food* is usually the most convenient scale of expression.

By resolution of the vitamin committee of the Health Organization of the League of Nations, the "International Unit of vitamin B_1" was set at three micrograms of the actual substance.

Sources of Thiamine

It is widely distributed in foods of both plant and animal origin. Plants synthesize thiamine. Though it occurs in various plant organs but is mainly present in mature dry seed. Brewer's yeast and wheat germ head the list of thiamine containing foods. The best sources of this in ordinary food are pork products, legumes, whole grains and enriched cereals. Nuts also contribute a lot of thiamine in food.

Riboplavin

As early as 1920, the belief that water soluble vitamin B was a single nutritive factor, was challenged and by about 1928 the fact had been definitely established that there were at least two vitamins contained in this complex, an antineuritic factor (vitamin B_1) now called thiamine and a growth promoting factor (vitamin G or B_2) now called riboflavin.

*Riboflavin*is the name, formally adopted by the American Medical Association, the Society of Biological Chemists, the American Institute of Nutrition, and the Federal Food and Drug Administration, and now in general use, for the water-soluble yellow substance with greenish fluorescence, which as isolated from milk is called lactoflavin.

Lactoflavin, ovoflavin, and *hepatoflavin* (all recognized as belonging to the group of organic substances known as flavins, and each named according to the natural source from which it was obtained) turned out to be identical, and the same substance became readily available as a synthetic product.

Its molecular structure and corresponding full name are shown in next page.

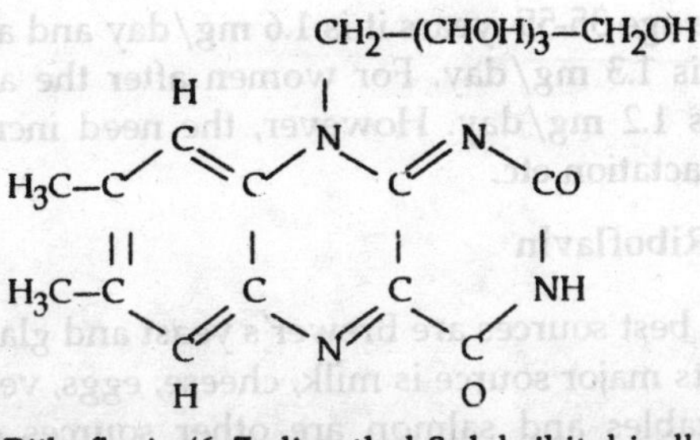

Fig. 10.4. Riiboflavin (6, 7, dimethyl-9-d, l-ribityl-isolloxazine).

Riboflavin is very widely distributed in both plant and animal tissues the so-called respiratory enzyme (Warburg's yellow enzyme) is combination of riboflavin phosphate with proteins.

The fact that riboflavin has been identified in such diverse products of life as milk, eggs, many microorganisms, liver, muscles, eyes, leaves, flowers, fruit, and seeds, and in both freshwater and saltwater algae, raises the presumption that it is almost if not quite universally involved in the life processes of active cells.

In milk, the riboflavin exists partly as an analogous compound.

Riboflavin occurs in yellow orange crystals, slightly soluble in water. The solutions of vitamin have a yellowish-green fluorescence. The presence of acids, heat and air have no destructive effect an vitamin but it is easily destroyed by alkalies and light.

Functions

It serves as a conenzyme is several of the enzyme systems of the body that are involved in the metoblism of the energy nutrients.

It is essential to growth and to normal nutrition at all levels. A deficiency of Riboflavin results in digestive disturbances, nervous, depression, general weakness, deterioration of tone and poor condition of eyes and skin. It reduces vitality, shortens life and aging process is faster.

A diet of higher riboflavin value results in better development, higher adult vitality greater freedom from disease at all ages, some what longer life.

Riboflavin has also been found to increase hemoglobin production in dogs.

Recommended Allowances of Riboflavin

For an adult (18-35 years) the suggested allowance of riboflavin is 1.7 mg /day for men and 1.3 mg /day for women.

Between the age 35-55 years it is 1.6 mg/day and above the age 55 years it is 1.3 mg/day. For women after the age of 35 it is proposed as 1.2 mg/day. However, the need increases during pregnancy lactation etc.

Sources of Riboflavin

Though best sources are Brewer's yeast and glandular meats but in diet its major source is milk, cheese, eggs, veal, beef, leafy green vegetables and salmon are other sources of riboflavin. Riboflavin values of same foods are fisted in Table 10.4.

Table 10.4. Riboflavin Values of Some Typical Foods

Food	*mg/100 gm*	*Portion*	*mg/Serving*
Brewer's yeast	4.28	1 tbsp	0.34
Liver, beef, cooked	4.19	2 oz	2.37
Heart, beef, cooked	1.22	3 oz	1.04
Cheese, Cheddar	0.46	1 oz	0.08
Egg	0.28	1 med	0.14
Veal roast, cooked	0.25	3 oz	0.26
Turnip greens, cooked	0.24	2/3 c	0.24
Beef, ground, cooked	0.21	3 oz	0.18
Bread, white, enriched	0.21	1 sl	0.04
Broccoli, cooked	0.20	2/3 c	0.20
Asparagus, cooded	0.18	2/3 c	0.21
Milk, whole	0.17	1 c	0.42
Salmon, canned	0.16	3 oz	0.16
Spinach, cooked	0.14	2/3 c	0.17
Bread, whole-wheat	0.12	1 sl	0.03
Bread, white, unenriched	0.09	1 sl	0.02
Orange juice, frozen	0.01	1 c	0.03
Butter	0	1 tbsp	0
Sugar, white	0	1 tsp	0

NIACIN (Nicotinic acid)

The disease, *pellagra*, which is now known to be prevented by an adequate body supply of Niacin, has been known for centuries.

The disease was considered to be associated with dietaries in which corn is a major staple food. It was not until 1930's that the pellagra-preventive factor in food was identified. It was in 1938 when Elvehjem et. al. were able to cure black tongue in dogs with nicotinamide isolated from liver, *nicotinic acid* was firmly established as pellagra-preventive factor.

Nicotinic acid is pyridine-3-carboxylic acid.

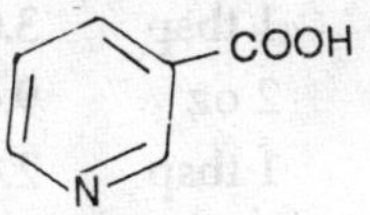

Nicotimic acid

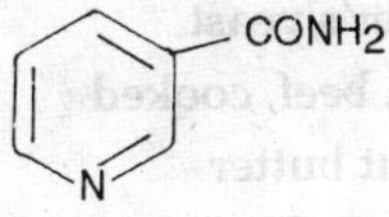

Nicotinamide

Nicotinic acid is a white crystalline compound as is easily converted to physiologically active compound, Nicotinamide.

Functions of Niacin

Like thiamine and riboflavin it acts as a constituent in coenzymes. It is a constituent of two coenzymes that are essential for certain oxidation reactions to occur in the body. One of the chief functions of coenzymes is the removal of hydrogen from certain compounds and transfer of it to others in a series of complex reactions.

Due to lack of niacin only dog develops characteristic deficiency symptoms other animals show symptoms such as reduced growth, loss of appetite, weight loss etc. The dog slows severe lesions of mouth, characteristic halitosis, diarrhea, emaciation and lack of appetite for food and water.

In man its deficiency causes pellagra. The early development of pellagra on corn diet is due to low digestibility of corn and low availability of niacin in corn.

Recommended Allowances of Niacin

NRC has recommended daily allowance is 19 mg equivalents of niacin (18-35 years), 17 mg equivalents (35-55 years) and 15 mg equivalents for older people. In case of women the recommended allowance is 14 mg equivalents (18-35 years) and 13 mg equivalents above 35 years of age.

Food Sources of Niacin

It occurs in both plant and animal products. The brewers yeast and peanut butter are best food sources. Table 10.5 lists the Niacin Values of same Foods.

Table 10.5. Niacin Values of Some Typical Foods

Food	*mg/100 gm*	*Portion*	*mg/Serving*
Brewer's yeast	37.9	1 tbsp	3.0
Liver, beef, cooked	16.5	2 oz	9.4
Peanut butter	15.7	1 tbsp	2.4
Chicken, Broiler, cooked	8.8	3 oz	7.4
Heart, beef, cooked	7.6	3 oz	6.5
Bran flakes, 40 per cent	6.2	1 oz	1.7
Beef, ground, cooked	5.4	3 oz	5.1
Almonds, shelled	3.5	1 c	5.0
Cornmeal, enriched, dry	3.5	1 c	5.1
Haddock, cooked	3.2	3 oz	2.7
Bread, whole-wheat	2.8	1 sl	0.7
Bread, white, enriched	2.4	1 sl	0.5
Peas, green, cooked	2.3	2/3 c	2.5
Potatoes, mashed	1.0	1 c	2.0
Tomato juice	0.8	1 c	1.8
Orange juice, frozen	0.3	1 c	0.8
Egg	0.1	1 med	trace
Milk, whole	0.1	1 c	0.1
Butter	0.0	1 tbsp	0
Sugar, white	0.0	1 tsp	0

Coffee is another important source of Niacin. In 100 gm of coffee there is about 10 mg of niacin.

10.8. Vitamin C (Ascorbic Acid)

Although man has known for years that the use of certain kinds of foods in his diet would prevent the occurrence of the disease, *Scurvy*, it was not until 1933 that Waugh and king at the university of Pittsburgh and Szent-Gyorgyi in Hungary identified the antiscurvy factor as ascorbic acid.

Ascorbic acid is the chemical name for vitamin C

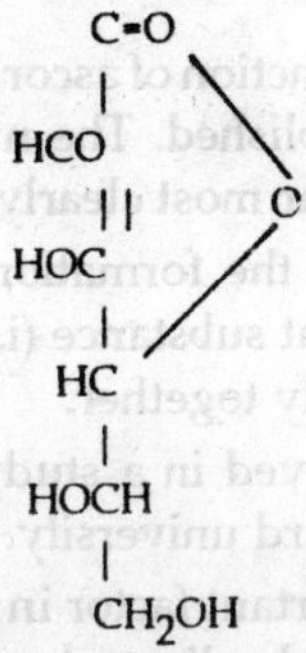

Fig. 10.5. Vitamin C (Ascorbic Acid): 2, 3 dienol-l-gulonic acid lactone.

It is a white crystalline substance soluble in water. The aqueous solution undergoes destruction on exposure to air, heat, light or metals like copper or iron. It is unstable in alkaline medium but stable in acid medium.

Until the decade, just one form of the vitamin, L-ascorbic acid (also called reduced ascorbic acid) was recognized as giving vitamin protection to man. Now, however, another form of the vitamin has been found that can be used as well as the reduced form. It has been named *dehydroascorbic* acid. The sum of the vitamin effect from both reduced and dehydroascorbic acids is referred to as *total* ascorbic acid. Experiments, conducted to determine how efficiently college students were able to utilize the total ascorbic acid from twenty-four different fruits and vegetables, have shown that the dehydroascorbic acid was used as well as the reduced form. Another chemical form of the vitamin, *erythorbic acid* (D-araboascorbic acid) is sometimes used as an antioxidant in food processing. This form, however, is only slightly antiscorbutic as compared to L-ascorbic acid.

The oxidation-reduction potential of ascorbic acid is such that it is reversibly oxidized to dehydroascorbic acid by a side variety of organic compounds and of inorganic reagents.

Among the former are the indophenol dyes, and among the latter is iodine. Both these have been employed quantitatively for the determination of ascorbic acid, in many plant and animal tissues including foods.

The method most generally adopted is that depending upon the carefully controlled oxidation of ascorbic acid to dehydroascorbic acid by the phenol-indophenol dye with the corresponding reduction of the latter to its leucobase, as developed by Bessey and King and modified for still greater accuracy.

Functions of Ascorbic Acid

The exact biochemical function of ascorbic acid in animals and men has not yet been established. The nutritional functions of vitamin C that has been so far most clearly established are:

(*i*) its relationship to the formation and maintenance of intercellular cement substance (i.e. collagen) that holds the cells of the body together.

This role was first observed in a study using a guinea pigs that was conducted at Harvard university.

Collagen is also an important factor in the process of healing of cuts or wounds. In wound healing when the intake of ascorbic acid is less than normal, it can be demonstrated that wounds do not heal normally. It has been demonstrated in connective tissue studies that ascorbic acid is essential for the production of tissue to enhance immediate postoperative healing and for the maintenance of previously formed scar tissue. Moreover the vitamin accumulates in scar tissue immediately following wounding and persists for a long period of time.

Three of the symptoms of scurvy that can be directly related to the loss of the cementing action of collagen are the hemorrhages that take place throughout the body, the loosening of the teeth, and the changes in the cells that occur in the extremities of the long bones of children and young animals. There is no doubt at the present time that a deficiency of ascorbic acid is directly related to poor collagen formation in the body, but the biochemical function of the vitamin in this reaction is still unknown.

(ii) its significance is safe guarding of the body through the blood;

(iii) its role in regulating the rate of cellular respiration.

Sealock has shown that ascorbic acid is essential for normal metabolism of the amino acid tyrosine in guinea pigs.

A relationship between ascorbic acid and the oxidation of the amino acid, tyrosine, has been observed in guinea pigs and infants but not in adult man. In scorbutic guinea pigs and infants it has been demonstrated that tyrosine is not metabolized normally unless sufficient ascorbic acid is available. In adults, however, this relationship was not observed when subjects were fed small amounts of the vitamin and large amounts of the amino acid. The role that ascorbic acid may play in the metabolism of tyrosine appears to be that of a coenzyme.

The cortical tissue of the adrenal glands contains a high concentration of ascorbic acid. Here, too, are found large amounts of cholesterol, the proposed parent substance of the cortical hormones. Tracer studies indicate that the vitamin may be involved in the conversion of acetate to cholesterol. However, the relationship of ascorbic acid to the cortical function of the adrenals has not yet been fully explained.

At present there is no conclusive evidence that the common cold, hay fever, and other related disorders can be prevented by high doses of ascorbic acid.

The Effects of an Ascorbic Acid Deficiency

In Animals: **The only animals other than man that have a** dietary need for ascorbic acid are guinea pigs and primates (monkeys, apes, chimpanzees). Other animals need the vitamin but they are able to synthesize enough ascorbic acid in their body tissues to meet the requirement.

Guinea pigs having leser intake of vitamin C showed loss of appetite, dull and rough hair etc. Sometimes it may result in hemorrhages.

In Man

Wolbach (1937) has especially emphasized the relation of this vitamin to the body's intercellular material. He points out that shortage of vitamin C may thus become the underlying cause: (1) of hemorrhages which may occur anywhere in the body; (2) of profound changes in the structure of the teeth and gums; (3) of changes in the growing ends of the bone with beading and other deformities which formerly were mistaken for rickets; (4) of the falling apart of bones due to loss of supporting cartilages (5) of enlargement of the heart and damage of heart muscles; (6) of degeneration of muscle fibers generally, causing extreme weakness and even death; (7) of the anemia due to destruction of blood-forming cells in the bone narrow and loss of blood by hemorrhage (8) of loss of calcium through degeneration of the bone matrix the bones sometimes becoming so soft that they break spontaneously; and (9) of a degeneration of the sex organs other glandular tissues.

Evidently then, vitamin C, the antiscorbutic substance, is much broader in its functioning than simply to prevent scurvy. When scurvy shall have been banished into ancient history, people will doubtless continue to study the functioning of vitamin C.

The absence of scurvy does not prove that the food is supplying as much vitamin C as the body needs for its best health, vigor, and ability to resist disease. Thus in the experiments of King and Menten (1935) in which guineapigs on graded levels of vitamin C intake received injections of graded amount of diphtheria toxin, it was demonstrated that the animals less liberally supplied with the vitamin, although they showed no external symptoms of scurvy, were much more sensitive to injury from the bacterial toxin at all dosages of the latter than were parallel animals on higher intakes of vitamin C.

Vitamin C probably functions in the nutritional processes of all species; those which do not need to have it in the food presumably make their own within their bodies.

Vitamin C Requirements in Human Nutrition: The Problem of adequate and Optimal Intakes

A daily intake of 25 milligrams of vitamin C by normal adults (other than women in pregnancy and lactation who need decidedly more) or 1.0 milligron per 100 calories o f food in family dietaries, might be regarded as a *minimum* sufficing for prevention of the gross signs of scurvy.

The Recommended Daily Allowances of the National Research Council's Food and Nutrition Board are: Men (average sized, regardless of activity), 75 mg.; Women (average sized, regardless of activity), 70 mg.; pregnancy (latter half), 100 mg.; lactation,150 mg.; Children, under 1 year, 30 mg.; 1-3 years, 35 mg.; 4-6 years, 50 mg.; 7-9 years, 60 mg.; 10-12 years, 75 mg.; Girls, 13-15 years, 80 mg 16-20 years, 80 mg; Boys, 13-15 years, 90 mg.; 16-20 years, 100 mg.

In 1963 revision the recommended daily allowance suggests that all individuals over the age 18 years need about 70 mg of vitamin C. An additional 30 mg has been proposed for the periods of pregnancy and lactation.

Food Source of Vitamin C

Fruits and vegetables are the main sources of ascorbic acid in diets. Citrus fruits (oranges, grapes, lemons and limes), berries

melons, tropical fruits (pine apple, guavas), leafy green vegetables, broccoli, green pepper, cabbage and tomatoes are good sources of vitamin C. Potatoes also are considered as a good source of vitamin C in diet.

Table 10.6. Vitamin C (Ascorbic Acid) in Certain Foods: Milligrams per 100 Grams of the Edible Portion

Food	*Range within which Final Average will Probably be Found*
Apples, medium varieties	5-8
Bananas	6-10
Cabbage, raw	29-52
Cantaloupe	26-35
Grapefruit	37-41
Kale	115-136
Lemons	50-56
Orange (or juice)	49-56
Peas, fresh young green, raw	22-26
Potatoes	14-20
Strawberries	34-60
Tomato (or fresh juice)	22-24
Turnips	25-30
Turnip greens	115-136
Watermelon	6-7

Mature, resting seeds contain practically no vitamin C. But if *properly sprouted grain or legume* be fed it is found to have considerable antiscorbutic value.

Frozen, concentrated orange juice amply deserves, and is receiving, widespread acclaim as an excellent antiscorbutic of high acceptability.

Hammer, Bernstein and Maynard (1945) have found that the greatest influence on ascorbic acid content of tomatoes was that of variations in light intensity to which the fruits are exposed previous to harvest.

Vitamin C is readily changed by oxidation and the greater part of the oxidation occurs upon heating under ordinary conditions.

More of vitamin C is destroyed when soda is added while cooking.

The vitamin C content of frozen fruits and vegetables has observed to be affected by changes in storage time and storage temperature. Marked loss is observed when stored longer than 4 months at + 10 °F.

Canned fruits are also subject to marked losses in ascorbic acid when stored at elevated temperatures for longer times.

A raw food has more vitamin C than the cooked one. The removal of the natural skin of a vegetable will increase the loss of vitamin C from food due to leaching of nutrient into the soaking or cooking water.

Cooking method used also can bring about a loss of vitamin C.

11

Water

11.1. Introduction

Water is by for the most critical of all nutrients. However, it is generally over looked when the nutrient needs of the body are enumerated. Animals will succumb to water deprivation sooner than to starvation. One can liver without food for about a month, but without water can not live for only a few days.

Water is an essential constituent of all cell structures and is the medium in which all the chemical reactions of cellular metabolism take place. Just as the life of one celled organism 'epends upon contact with its watery environment for sustenance, the cells of higher organisms are dependent upon the aqueous medium within and surrounding cell structures. Water makes up approximately 65% of the body weight. The total volume of water is related to the mass of lean tissues of the body rather than to the body weight. Fat tissue contains less water than lean tissues.

Approximately two-thirds of the water content of the body is contained within the cells (intracellular fluid), and the remaining one-third is found in spaces outside the cell (extracellular fluid). The extracellular fluid consists of the fluid between tissues and cells (interstitial fluid) and the water present in the blood plasma. Between 3 to 4 qt of water circulates in the blood stream.

11.2. Functions of Water

Various functions performed by water in animal body include such functions as follows. It acts as

(i) a building material,

(ii) a solvent,

(*iii*) a lubricant, and

(*iv*) a temperature regulator.

As a *building material* water is used in construction of every cell. Just as the life of one called organism depends upon contact with its watery environment for sustenance, the cells of higher organisms are dependent upon the aqueous medium within and surrounding cell structures. The cells and tissues of body however vary in their water content. For example, dentin contains 10% water, fatty tissues 20%, bone 25% and striated muscles 80%.

As a *solvent,* water is essential for the normal functioning of body cells. Water is compatible with more substances than any other known solvent, and therefore it is an ideal medium for transporting nutrients to the tissue cells and in which the chemical reactions of cellular metabolism can take place. Its role however is, more than that of a passive reaction medium. In hydrolytic and hydration reactions water is an active participant in body metabolism. Water is used in digestive processes where it acids in the mastication and softening of food, supplies fluid for the digestive juices, and facilitates the movement of the food mass along the digestive tract. After digestion the nutrients, in a state of solution or suspension, pass through the intestinal wills and are carried away by either the blood or the lymph. In the cells water is the fluid medium where in the intercellular chemical reactions occur. After metabolism the blood, which is about 92% water, picks up the waste products from the cells and carries them either to the lungs or kidneys for excretion.

Water serves as a *lubricant* in the joints and between internal organs. It bathes the body cells, keeping them moist and permitting the passage of substances between the cells and the blood vessels.

As a *regulator of body temperature* water aids in the removal of heat from the body. The regulation of body temperature is dependent partially upon the conductivity property of water to distribute heat evenly within the body and eventually to remove by vaporization the excess heat released by metabolic reactions within the body cells. The evaporation of water on the skin surface is an effective way of eliminating generated body heat. Approximately 1 qt of perspiration dissipates 580 Cal of heat. However, during strenuous physical activity or in a hot dry atmosphere the loss of moisture by skin evaporation may be markedly increased. A football player loses about 10-12 pounds of body weight during a game. This loss is mostly as a loss of water through sweating Drastic changes in body temperature are however prevented by other properties of water, such as high specific heat and high latent heat of vapourisation. Thus more heat is required to change water from liquid to vapour or liquid to solid than any other substances. These properties alone establish water as a superior medium for metabolic activities. Sudden and violent changes in body temperature obviously would disrupt the enzymatic machinery or the animal cell.

11.3. Sources of Water for the Body

The water auxilable to the animal body includes the water present in liquid and solid food consumed and water formed in cells because of the oxidation of food stuffs. This endogenous water is called metabolic water or water of oxidation. Metabolic water amounts to about 15% of the daily total water available from an ordinary in take of foods and drinks. The water of oxidation has been computed for various food stuffs by Newburgh (1930) and Peters (1933). The figures vary slightly for carbohydrate and protein, as shown below:

Food stuff	*Water of oxidation (in gm)*	
(100 grams)	*Newburgh*	*Peters*
Protein	41	40
Carbohydrates	60	56
Fats	107	107

Thus, the total amount of water available to the body can be calculated if we know the composition of the diet as well as the consumption of other beverages. The largest amount of water comes from ingested fluids. The average person consumes approximately 1-1.5 qt. of fluid as water, coffee, tea, soup and other liquids each day.

The water content of foods varies widely, with most foods in the average diet containing more than 70% moisture. The percentage of water in some common food items are shown in Fig 11.1.

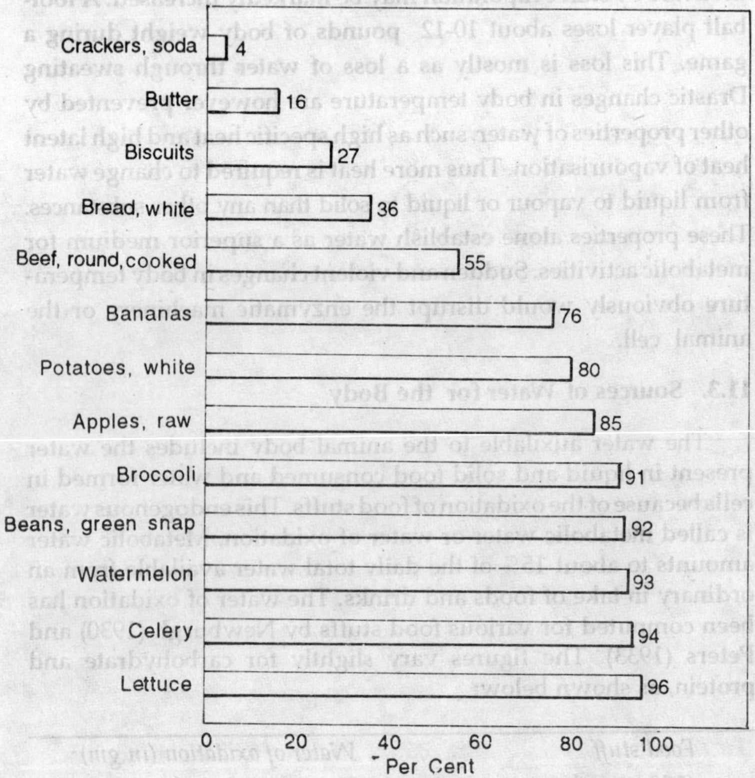

Fig. 11.1. Percentage of water in some commonly used foods.

11.4. Excretion of Water from the Body

Water is lost from the body by way of kidneys (urine), skin (perspiration), lungs (expired air), intestinal canal (feces) and eyes (tears). The amount of water lost by the body is influenced by water intake, body conditions, and environmental conditions. The maximum water loss occurs through kidneys (urine). The excretion of urine is greatly influenced by fluid in take. The amount excreted by skin (perspiration) varies according to the need for the body to lose heat to regulate body temperature.

When an individual is physically or the environmental temperature is high, proportionately more water will be lost through the skin than under normal conditions. Insensible perspiration is usually not noticed because each area gives off such a small amount; however, a pint a day is usually lost by this means.

An example of the water balance of an individual is given in Table 11.1.

Table 11.1. Water Balance (Average Individual)

Water Intake	Milliters
Liquid food (water, coffee, milk, soup)	1100
Solid food (moisture)	500–900
Water of oxidation	400
	2000–2400
Water Output	
Vaporization (400 ml expired as moist air—lung, and 600 ml skin sweat)	920–1000
Feces	80–100
Urine	1000–1300
	2000–2400

The excessive water loss from the body, as in profuse sweating, diarrhea, or prolonged episodes of vomiting results in dehydration and in loss of electrolytes. The danger of replenishing the body water without concurrent repletion of electrolytes leads to water intoxications. Symptoms of dehydration may occur when 5-10% of body water has been lost. The symptoms of dehydration are thirst, dryness of mouth, feeling of weakness, and increased pulse rate. Dehydration may be overcome by the use of water, water and salt or water + minerals.

11.5. Recommended Allowance for Water

According to NRC the standard for calculating the daily water allowance is 1 mg par kcal of food. Individuals satisfying the thirst or the desire for water is the only criterion necessary to meet the body's need. Under conditions of extreme heat where there is excessive sweating, the thirst mechanism may not allow for the drinking of sufficient water, making it necessary to supplement the natural intake. Five or six glasses of fluids should be consumed daily as water or in beverage. The habit of drinking water should be encouraged because water is important to normal functioning of the body. Water consumption at meal time is advised if the food is properly masticated, not if water is not used to wash down the food. Water is thought to aid digestion by promoting the flow of digestive juices.

12

Nutritional Aspects of Acid-Base Balance

12.1. Introduction

Though a large amount of various acids are produced during metabolic reactions in the body but the reaction of the blood plasma remains fairly constant and slightly alkaline (ranges between pH = 7.33 to pH =7.51). In case of healthy individuals some departure from this normal range in noticed, during forced breathing or strenuous exercise, for short periods of time. However the extreme ranges reported is pH = 7.0 to 7.8.

12.2. Buffers of the Blood

All body fluids have pH values which must be maintained within relatively narrow limits and with in which the cells function normally. These pH values are not the same in every part of the body, for example the pH of some secretions are given below:

Blood	7.4 to 7.5
Bile	7.8 to 8.6
Pancreatic juice	8.0
Saliva	6.4 to 6.8
Urine	5.5 to 7.0
Gastric juice	1.5 to 1.8

pH of a solution is defined as the negative logarithms to the base 10 of the hydrogen ion cencentration. Thus

$$pH = -\log [H^+] = \log \frac{1}{[H^+]}$$

The pH of blood normally is 7.4 or $[H^+]$ = 40 nanomoles per litre.

The pH scale runs from 1 to 14. A solution having pH between 0 and 7 is acidic and a solution having pH between 7 and 14 is basic in nature. The acidic or basic nature of the environment has a profound effect on the cells and so the maintenance of normal hydrogen ion concentration within the body is an important factor in the environment of the cells.

Buffers refers to such solutions which do not show any change in their pH when a small quantity of acid or alkali is added to them. This is because such solutions have the capability to "bind" hydrogen ion or hydroxye ion without change in pH.

The buffer may be acidic or basic in nature. The pH of acidic buffers lies in the range 0-7 and those of basic buffer in the range 7-14.

In animals we find three major buffer systems. These are—

(i) Phosphate system

(ii) Bicarbonate system, and

(iii) Amino acid system.

Blood is a highly buffered system and it is because of this that it can receive such large quantities of acidic products formed by the cells without any change in its "reaction".

The most important buffer system of blood are those of the proteins and their alkali salts. The proteins are amphoteric in nature so they are capable of acting either as acid or as a base.

Since chief proteins of the blood have isoelectric points more acids than the natural medium in which each occurs, they are presumably present at this hydrogen ion activity as buffer systems made up of proteins in its acid form (HP),with an excess of its alkali salt (BP). Van slyke states that about one-tenth of the buffer power of the blood is attributable to the plasma protein, much the greater part of the remainder being due to hemoglobin. This is due to the higher concentration of the latter (human blood contains in 100 cc about 15-16 g hemoglobin and 3.5 to 4.0 gram plasma protein) but also because at the hydrogen ion concentration of blood, the *buffer value* of hemoglobin is more than twice as great as that of plasma protein.

Hastings and Eisele (1940) found the acid-base balance of the blood of a normal adult at rest "to vary (in a regular, not random manner) during a 24-hours period due to....*(a)* a rise in the plasma HCO_3 associated with the intestine of food; *(b)* an increase in the CO_2 tension of the blood associated with sleep."

Phosphate Systems

Phosphates in the blood form buffer mixtures made up of the acid ($H^+ B^+ HPO_4^=$) ant its salts ($B^+ B^+ HPO_4^=$). A buffer system is most effective at a hydrogen ion activity approximating the dissociation constant of the buffer acid. Since the dissociation constant (pK) of monobasic phosphate at physiological salt concentrations is about 6.8, the reaction of the plasma is favourable for the buffer activity of the phosphates. However, their concentration in the blood is so low that their buffer effect here is overshadowed by that of the proteins.

A solution of sodium dihydrogen phosphate ionizes in solution as under:

$$NaH_2PO_4 \rightleftharpoons Na^+ + H_2PO_4^- \rightleftharpoons H^+ + HPO_4^{2-} \rightleftharpoons H^+ + PO_4^{3-}$$

The final ionization in the above sequence is only half complete at a pH of about 13.0, and so can be ignored from a physiological point of view. The predominant phosphate ions in solution at a physiological pH will therefore be $H_2PO_4^-$ and HPO_4^{2-}. Phosphate buffers in fact, are usually made up as a mixture of two salts, sodium dihydrogen phosphate, NaH_2PO_4, and disodium hydrogen phosphate, Na_2HPO_4. It is evident from the scheme of ionization given above that the second of these two salts act as a weak acid as it produce same hydrogen ions in solution, where as the first salt represents the salt of phosphoric acid H_3Po_4 with strong base Na OH. The mixture of these two salts will behave as a buffer. Thus if hydrogen ions are added, water is formed.

$$NaH_2PO_4 + NaOH \rightarrow Na_2HPO_4 + H_2O$$

The addition of acid results in the formation of basic salt.

$$Na_2HPO_4 + HCL \rightarrow NaCl + NaH_2PO_4.$$

Elimination of Carbonic Acids

The bicarbonate-carbonic acid system has little buffer effects since, in solutions of the same ionic strength as blood plasma, the maximum buffer efficiency is observed at about pH 6.1, far from the pH of the plasma. Nevertheless, the blood bicarbonate has a special significance in the maintenance of a constant hydrogen ion activity with in the body, since, because its acid is volatile, the large store of base combined in this way is available for the neutralization of acids other than carbonic. On the other hand, any base which is present in excess of acids other than carbonic takes the form of bicarbonate. Because of these properties the bicarbonate of the blood has been called the *alkaline reserve.* It is considered by Peters and Van Slyke as reflecting more or less closely the reserve of available alkali present in the body as a whole.

The bicarbonate buffer system ($H_2CO_3 - HCO_3^-$) has same characteristic features. While it functions as a buffer in the same manner as other conjugate acid base pairs, the h_K of H_2CO_3, a relatively strong acid, is about 3.8 which is much lower than the normal range of blood pH. In bicarbonate buffer system, the protein- donor species carbonic acid is in reversible equilibrium with dissolved CO_2.

$$CO_2 \text{ dissolved} \rightleftharpoons CO_2 \text{ (gas)}$$

Since according to Henry's law the solubility of a gas in water is proportional to its partial pressure, the pH of the bicarbonate buffer system is a function of the partial pressure of CO_2 in the gas phase over the buffer solution. If the CO_2 pressure is increased, all other variable remaining constant, the pH of the bicarbonate buffer decreases, and vice versa. The bicarbonate buffer can buffer effectively near pH = 7.0, at which the protein acceptor /proton donor ratio is very high, since a small quantity of proton donor H_2CO_3 is in labile equilibrium with a relatively large reserve capacity of gaseous CO_2 in the lungs. Under the conditions in which the blood must absorb excess OH^-; the H_2CO_3 which is used up and converted to HCO_3^- is quickly replaced from the large pool of CO_2 (gaseous) in the lungs.

There is another characteristic feature of the bicarbonate buffer system. CO_2 is the end product of the aerobic combustion of fuel molecules in the vertebrate and is ultimately expired from the lungs. The steady-state ratio of $\frac{[HCO_3^-]}{[H_2CO_3]}$ in the blood is a reflection of the rate of CO_2 production during tissue oxidation and of the rate of less of CO_2 by expiration.

Thus of the acids which, in the normal process of metabolism, are continually formed in the cells, carbon dioxide is quantitatively by far the most prominent. The means by which it is transported from the cells to the lungs to be eliminated, without marked change in the hydrogen ion activity of the blood, are of special interest. To some extent, carbonic acid, like any other acid, is neutralized by the blood buffer systems which have been discussed. In addition, hemoglobin is rather uniquely adapted to function as a carrier of carbon dioxide as well as of oxygen. In the lungs, where the oxygen tension is high, hemoglobin combines readily with oxygen to form oxygenated hemoglobin; this is turn gives up its oxygen when it reaches the tissues, where the oxygen tension is low. Since the oxygenated form is distinctly stronger acid than the reduced form, the change in the state of oxidation of hemoglobin which occurs at the tissues is similar to the removal of acid. Less base being required to neutralize the weaker acid (reduced hemoglobin), more is made available to react with the increased amount of carbonic acid which is being received simultaneously by the blood. On the other hand, at the lungs, where hemoglobin is reoxygenated, the effect upon the bicarbonate of the blood is similar to the addition of acid, and results in an increased formation of carbon dioxide which is excreted.

Conversely, the tendency to increased activity resulting from the higher tension of carbon dioxide in the tissues causes an increase in the dissociation of oxygenated hemoglobin into oxygen and hemoglobin, i.e., tends of increase the liberation of oxygen in the tissues. Thus, the formation of oxygenated hemoglobin in the lungs directly increases the excretion of carbon dioxide while the increased tension of carbon dioxide in the tissues increases the liberation of oxygen from combination with hemoglobin.

Roughton and others have stressed the possibility that hemoglobin may combine chemically with carbon dioxide, the compound (or compounds) thus formed, *carbhemoglobin,* aiding significantly in the carrying of carbon dioxide in the blood.

Another constituent of the red blood cells, an enzyme (*carbonic anhydrase*) which accelerates the dehydration of carbonic acid to carbon dioxide and the reverse conversion of carbon dioxide to carbonic acid, assists in the interchange of gases both in the lungs and in the tissues.

From the forgoing discussion, it becomes clear that the cells of the blood are richly buffered; whereas the plasma, is only poorly buffered. Van Slyke and his coworkers have shown, that, under physiological conditions, the buffering ability of the cells is shared with the plasma by an exchange of ions called the *chloride shift.* There is also evidence that other anions to which the cell membranes are permeable, such as sulfate and phosphate, may undergo a similar redistribution with changing concentrations of carbon dioxide, but their influence is relatively slight because of their much lower concentration.

Another important factors in the elimination of carbon dioxide and in the regulation of the acid-base balance of the body is the fact that there is a tendency for the respiratory process to hold the tension of carbon dioxide in the blood nearly constant. Both the depth and the frequency of breathing are supposed to be under the control of the so-called *respiratory centres* in the brain, the activity of which is most directly influenced by the pH of the cells in the centre (Gesell, 1925). An increased production of carbon dioxide because of accelerated metabolism, during exercise, for example, tends to lower the pH of the blood, and so, of the cells in the respiratory centre. This change stimulates breathing so that more carbon dioxide is eliminated by the lungs, and the hydrogen ion activity and the carbon dioxide tension of the blood are restored toward normal. According to Henderson (1928), "it is the changing ventilation of the lungs that most directly controls the acid-base equilibrium of the blood."

Elimination of Fixed Acids

Fixed acids are non-volatile and their elimination involves two main steps.

(i) the immediate reaction of the acids with the bicarbonates and buffer salts of the blood or tissues;

(ii) the subsequent elimination of these acids as salts by the kidneys.

The action of bicarbonates and buffers of the blood in centralizing these acids immediately as they are formed is indeed a most important safeguard for the organism. However, it is only a temporary measure, because the salt of the fixed acids formed in this way remain to be excreted and their removal from the blood involves the simultaneous removal of basic substances as well. In itself, this would tend to reduce the bicarbonate concentration or the alkali reserve of the blood and this results in the loss of fixed base from the body. It is here that ammonia and the buffer action of the salts of the urine play an important role.

The kidneys is capable of forming ammonia, that combines with the acid to be excreted, replacing in part the fixed bases, which latter are returned to the blood in the form of bicarbonates. The quantity of ammonia so produced varies directly with the quantity of fixed acid to be excepted; and thus is derived from glutamine and, to a lesser extent, from amino acids.

In contrast to that of the blood, the hydrogen ion activity of the urine varies rather widely, from about pH 4.8 to about pH 8.4, depending upon the proportions of acid and basic products formed in metabolism and upon the amounts and proportions of these products which are removed from the blood through other channels (particularly the lungs and the gastrointestinal tract). Strong acids like hydrochloric and sulfuric cannot exist as such, to any appreciable extent, in solutions of the hydrogen ion activity of the urine and must therefore be excreted with their chemical equivalent of base. On the other hand, weaker acids, like monobasic phosphate and some of the organic acids of the urine, act as effective buffers in acid urine, an increased acidity of the urine resulting in the excretion of a larger fraction of the buffer in the acid form. For example, at pH 7.4 in the blood, about 80% of the total inorganic phosphate is in the dibasic form, while at pH 4.8 in extremely acid urine, about 1% is in the dibasic form, the remainder being in the monobasic form. In other words, by excreting a urine of pH 4.8, the body is able to conserve about two fifths of the base which had been combined in the blood with the excreted phosphate.

The acids which are constantly added to the tissue fluids by the cells are first buffered and then disposed in various ways. Lactic acid formed from muscular contraction is partly converted back into glycogen by the liver. Phosphates, sulfates and chlorides are excreted by the kidneys. Carbon dioxide which is continentally produced by all cells, is removed in the lungs which thus exert an accurate and rapid control over the acid-base balance.

Excretion of Organic Acids

In rare cases when there is a temporary loss of acid (e.g. during active gastric secretion) the kidney helps in the maintenance of constant $[H^+]$ within the body. The urine becomes alkaline and so the phosphate combines with relatively more fixed base. The excretion of ammonia practically ceases, fixed base being used instead for the neutralization of organic and in organic acids. A large part of the excess base is eliminated as bicarbonate. The organic acids of the urine are of practically no significance as *buffers* under these conditions, since at the pH of the blood they exist almost wholly as neutral salts, and consequently can combine with little more base even at a more alkaline pH. In certain cases of alkali excess there is increased formation and excretion of organic acids, these additional quantities of acids remove from the body, their equivalent fixed bases.

If has been found that the urinary excretion of citrate for any given individual tends to parallel closely from day to day pH of the urine, rising with an increase in alkalinity irrespective of the dietary change that was responsible for this increase. Under usually dietary conditions, the excretion of citric acid varies from about one quarter of a gram to one gram, but when sodium bicarbonate is taken by mouth, more than two grams of citrate may be present in the urine. Though the citric acid synthesized by body may be of some importance in conserving the fixed acids of the body when there is an excess of basic elements to be eliminated but the amount of base which is removed in combination with the organic acids when the urine is alkaline is only a small fraction of that which can be eliminated as bicarbonate.

Various acids found in human urine are listed below in Table 12.1.

Table 12.1. Organic Acids of Urine

Acid	*Dissociation Constant* K_a	*Normal Excretion Mg. per Day*
1	2	3
Citric	K_1 8.3×10^{-4} K_2 4.1×10^{-5} K_3 3.2×10^{-6}	200-1200
Uric	1.5×10^{-6}	200-1000
Hippuric	2.2×10^{-4}	100-1500
Lactic	1.3×10^{-4}	70-100

(contd.)

1	2	3
Formic	2.1×10^{-4}	10-100
Oxalic	3.8×10^{-2}	10-50
β-hydroxybutyric	3.9×10^{-5}	0-75

Influence of Diet

In certain cases when the proportions of fat, carbohydrate and protein are unbalanced in such a way that they upset the normal ketogenic-antiketogenic relationship then the body may be flooded with organic acids arising from incomplete oxidation of fat. In this state which is similar to a state found in cases of diabetic acidosis. This type of ketosis is quite common in starvation and is sometimes produced artificially by a ketogenic (high fat low carbohydrate) diet for therapeutic purposes. Such a situation is very rare in normal individuals on self-chosen diet.

Since the non-volatile end products of normal metabolism are almost entirely inorganic in nature (with the exception of urea, which is neutral in reaction), an approximate estimate of the potential acid or base-forming properties of a food may be made from a consideration of the amounts and proportions of the inorganic elements which it contains. A fairly large number of foods were analyzed and their balance of acid-forming and base-forming elements computed by Sherman and Gettler (1912). For this calculation, the amounts of chlorine, phosphorus, and sulfur present were expressed as the equivalent number of cubic centimeters of normal acids; the amounts of calcium, magnesium, potassium, and sodium present were expressed as the equivalent number of cubic centimeters of normal alkali; and the predominance of acid-forming or base- forming potential was obtained by difference. Typical results are shown in Tables 12.2 and 12.3.

Table 12.2. Examples of Foods in which Acid-forming Elements Predominate

Food (Edible Portion)	*Approximate Potential Acidity (cc. Normal Acid)*	
	Per 100 Grams	*Per 100 Calories*
1	2	3
Beef, clear lean	12	10
round steak	11	7

1	2	3
Eggs	11	7
Oatmeal	12	3
Oysters	15	30
Rice	9	2
Wheat, entire	12	3
Wheat flour	9	2
White bread, made with water	6	2

Table 12.3. Examples of Foods in which Base-formic Elements Predominate

Food (Edible Portion)	*Approximate Potential Reserve Alkalinity (cc. Normal Acid)*	
	Per 100 Grams	*Per 100 Calorics*
Apples	3	6
Bananas	8	8
Beans, dried	10	3
string, fresh	5	13
Beet, fresh	10	25
Cantaloupe	7	18
Carrots	14	30
Citron	9	3
Dates	9	3
Lemon or juice	4	10
Onions	1	2
Orange or juice	5	10
Pears, fresh	4	5
Potatoes	9	10
Radishes	5	23
Rutabagas	8	29
Sweetpotatoes	6	5
Tomatoes	5	24
Turnips	11	33
Watermelon	4	12

While making these calculations the following assumptions have been used.

(i) Phosphorus has been calculated as a dibasic acid.

(ii) Sulphur is completely oxidized and neutralized entirely by inorganic base.

(iii) Organic acids and carbon dioxide have not been taken into consideration for these calculations.

Inspite of these limitations, the results calculated from the mineral analyses of foods have in practice shown a general relationship to the effects of the foods on the acid-base balance of the body, as indicated by the urinary acidity and ammonia, except in those cases in which the food contains a considerable amount of some organic acid which is not oxidized in the body. The foods of which this is known to be true are omitted from the accompanying tables. The mineral contents of commercial fats, sugars, and starches are too low for these to have any significant effect upon the acid-base balance, so they also are omitted from these tables.

In their experiments on man, Sherman and Gettler have studied the effect of replacing the potato of a mixed diet by rice. It was found that 33% of the calculated increase of fixed acid from metabolism was accounted for by an increase in the urinary ammonia, and about 40% by the increased titratable acidity of the urine. The remainder of the excess fixed acid may have been eliminated, in part at least, through the skin or in feces, or may have been neutralized by the buffers of the blood with a corresponding increase in the carbon dioxide output and decrease in the reserve alkalinity of the body. In this experiment, the intake and output of phosphorus were approximately the same on the two diets. The increased acidity of the urine, therefore, implied an increased ratio of primary to secondary phosphate in the urine but not necessarily an increase in the amount of fixed base leaving the body. In the neutralization of sulfuric acid by means of phosphate, each molecule of the acid (representing one atom of sulfur oxidized to sulfate in protein metabolism) changes two molecules of secondary into primary phosphate. Whether or not this results in increased excretion of phosphate and therefore of fixed base (or only, as in the experiment just cited, in an altered ratio of primary and secondary phosphate in the urine) apparently depends upon a complex combination of conditions not yet fully understood.

Certain fruits and fruit juices have large amounts of organic acids, such as citric acid which is perhaps the most familiar. Most of these are di-or tribasic acids and exist in the fruits partly as potassium acid salts and partly as free acids. These fruits when eaten have an acid reaction; whether they are potentially acid or potentially basic in metabolism depends upon the extent to which the organic acid radicles are oxidized in the body, with the formation of potassium bicarbonate. Thus tomatoes, oranges, pears, peaches, apricots, and pineapples tend to lower the acidity of the urine, while, cranberries, plums, and prunes increase urinary acidity The behaviour of this latter group is due to the presence in these fruits of relatively large quantities of quinic acid, which, instead of being oxidized completely in the body, is converted into hippuric acid which appears in the urine. It has been found that when human beings take by mouth as much as forty grams of citric acid (more than it seem likely that they would ingest per day in their food), less than 5% of the acid appears in the urine (Sherman, Mendel, Smith and Toothill, 1936b). Very little is known of the fate of malic acid in the human organism, although cats, rabbits, and dogs can destroy it to a large extent. Human tissues apparently have almost no ability to oxidize tartaric acid. When tartrates or grape juice are taken by mouth, however, only a small fraction of the acid reappears in the excrete, the greater part being destroyed by the microorganisms in the gastrointestinal tract. The observation that the ingestion of grape products may, under favourable conditions, lower the urinary acidity can be explained by the absorption of potassium bicarbonate that is a probable end product of bacterial action on the potassium acid tartrate of the grape.

Oxalates are found in small quantities in a great many fruits and vegetables, and in very considerable quantities in certain plants, especially of the family Chenopodiaceae, including beet greens, chard, spinach and sorrel. Little is known about the ability of the body to metabolize oxalate. Moreover, the insolubility of calcium oxalate throughout the digestive tract makes it doubtful how much of the oxalic acid of the food is actually absorbed; and, conversely, oxalate in the food may greatly reduce the absorption of food calcium (Fincke and Sherman, 1935). Oxalic acid in small quantities is a normal constituent of the blood and urine, and probably, like citric acid, it is formed in metabolism.

Relatively little attention has yet been given to the important finding of Rous (1925) that all or most of the body tissues are somewhat less alkaline than the blood plasma, while the organs in which the nutritional processes are particularly active are, or may be, frankly acid (around pH 5.6). Thus some of the most important parts of the body get only partially the benefit of the buffering capacity of the blood, and so may be more influenced by an excess of acid-forming elements in the food than the studies of the blood would seem to suggest.

The working-out of the problems of the buffers and the carbonic acid carrying capacity of the blood is an outstandingly brilliant triumph of physico-chemical research. This knowledge of the blood, however, does not solve the problems of acid-base balance in all the separate organs of the body, nor permit one to say with confidence whether the balance of acid-forming and base-forming elements in food is or is not of practical significance in human nutrition.

13

Dietary Adequacy and Nutritional Status

13.1. Introduction

The word adequacy is ambiguous and Heilbron, Jones and Bacharach have pointed out that the quantities of vitamin A requirement just necessary to prevent overt signs of deficiency is definitely less than that required to maintain "normal health". Now it has been generally accepted that health is not merely the absence of disease but rather it is positive quality of life that can be built by degrees to successively higher levels.

Thus between the lowest level at which one can live and the much higher level of nutritional well-being to which alone the term *optimal* is properly applied, there is with some nutrients a highly significant field of gradual improvement which we can subdivide more or less elaborately into different degrees or levels or zones, depending in part upon the delicacy of our methods of discrimination and in part upon the nutrient factor with which we are dealing. This last is important to emphasize clearly, for it is quite unscientific to assume that the difference between minimal-adequate and optimal intake is equally important for all nutrient factors.

Each nutrient factor should be studied on its own merits in this respect. The difference between minimal-adequate and optimal intake may be less than 10% with calories and more than 100 per cent with calcium or vitamin A or C. And if there is good evidence of a very wide difference with one vitamin, this fact creates no presumption as to what that difference will prove to be with some other vitamins.

13.2. The Concept of Dietary Standards or Allowances in Chemical Terms

The first organized attempt at developing a dietary standard came as a result of food shortages during World War I when it became necessary for United States Government to devise a rational basis for shipments of food from that country to its allies in Europe.

In 1933, the British Medical Association proposed a limited set of standard and in the same year United States Department of Agriculture made more extensive proposals including recommendations for energy value, protein, calcium, iron, phosphorus, vitamin A and ascorbic acid.

The League of Nations Technical Commission on Nutrition focused international attention on the significance of diet in preventive medicine and as a means of improving the public health. Dietary standards were proposed for energy and protein expressed as an average requirement on the basis of age, sex and activity.

The National Research Council's Recommended Dietary Allowances aim to furnish guidance for the nourishment of the body at *desirable levels.* These as now conceived by the Food and Nutrition Board of the National Research Council are shown in Table 13.1.

The term *Recommended Allowances* was advisedly chosen after careful consideration of all suggest alternatives.

The data is intended to represent levels of nutritional intakes which are desirable goals.

The recommendations are not called "requirements" because they are intended to represent not merely the literal (minimal) requirements of average individuals, but "levels enough higher to cover substantially all individual variations in the requirements of normal people..."

Table 13.1. Recommended Daily Dietary Allowances[a] Food and Nutrition Board, National Research Council

	Calories	*Protein, Gm.*	*Cal-cium, Gm*	*Iron, Mg.*	*Vita-min A, I.U.*	*Thia-mine, Mg.*	*Ribo-flavin, Mg.*	*Niacin (Nicotinic acid), Mg.*	*Ascor-bic acid, Mg.*	*Vitamin D, I.U.*
Man (154 lb., 70 kg.)										
Sedentary	2400	70	1.0	12 *e*	5000	1.2	1.8	12	75	*f*
Physically active	3000	70	1.0	12 *e*	5000	1.5	1.8	15	75	*f*
With heavy work	4500	70	1.0	12 *e*	5000	1.8	1.8	18	75	*f*
Woman (124 lb., 56 kg.)										
Sedentary	2000	60	1.0	12	5000	1.0	1.5	10	70	*f*
Moderately active	2400	60	1.0	12	5000	1.2	1.5	12	70	*f*
Very active	3000	60	1.0	12	5000	1.5	1.5	15	70	*f*
Pregnancy (latter half)	2400	85	1.5	15	6000	1.5	2.5	15	100	400
Lactation	3000	100	2.0	15	8000	1.5	3.0	15	150	400
Children up to 12 yrs.	110/2.2 lb.	3.5/2.2 lb.								
Under 1 yr.	(1 kg.)	(1 kg.)	1.0	6	1500	0.4	0.6	4	30	400
1-3 yrs. (27 lb., 12 kg.)	1200	40	1.0	7	2000	0.6	0.9	6	35	400
4-6 yrs. (42 lb., 19 kg.)	1600	50	1.0	8	2500	0.8	1.2	8	50	400
7-9 yrs. (58 lb., 26 kg.)	2000	60	1.0	10	3500	1.0	1.5	10	60	400
10-12 yrs. (78 lb., 35 kg.)	2500	70	1.2	12	4500	1.2	1.8	12	75	400
Children over 12 yrs.										
Girls, 13-15 yrs. (108 lb., 49 kg.)	2600	80	1.3	15	5000	1.3	2.0	13	80	400
16-20 yrs. (122 lb., 55 kg.)	2400	75	1.0	15	5000	1.2	1.8	12	80	400
Boys 13-15 yrs. (108 lb., 49 kg.)	3200	85	1.4	15	5000	1.5	2.0	15	90	400
16-20 yrs. (141 lb., 64 kg.)	3800	100	1.4	15	6000	1.7	2.5	17	100	400

The term *minimum requirement* represents basic physiological need and is the smallest amount of a nutrient that will prevent deficiency symptom or support a well defined physiological or biochemical response.

The term *average requirement* is used to denote the amount of a nutrient that will support health in most persons and so it implies that the *true requirement* for individuals may be either above or below the average for the group.

Thus both the above terms are ambiguous and so the term requirement is avoided in dietary standards. *Allowances* is more accurate description and implies the addition of an amount above the estimated requirement to cover both the variation among individuals and the lack of precision inherent in the estimated requirement. This additional amount is the *safety factor* known as *margin of safety* or *allowance for safety.*

Now we have enough evidence to show that the margins between optimal intake and minimal requirements are wider for some nutrients than for others. More over nutrients may vary widely in respect to the desirability surplus intake.

"The usual undiscriminating view is that, if the diet furnishes enough of any given factor to meet functional need, any further amount supplied by the food is normally a matter very nearly of indifference, significant only as a sort of insurance against some emergency. This may be true for most of the essential food factors. Of a few nutrients, however, there is evidence that one may, in the course of a lifetime, derive increased benefit from increased intake up to levels very considerably above those of ordinarily accepted adequacy. (Ascorbic acid, vitamin A, and calcium are perhaps the best established cases of this kind.) Conversely, it may be true of some other nutrient factors that surplus intakes should be held within bounds if undesirable consequences are to be avoided. The outstanding and undisputed example of the latter is the energy value or calories of the diet, of which any considerable surplus intake tends to induce overweight."

Energy allowances for children may need adjustment some-what above or below the Recommended Allowances according to the size, build, and activity of the child. The ranges shown in Table 13.2 will probably cover ordinary cases.

Table 13.2. Food Allowances for Children of about Average Weight for their Age

Age Years	*Calories Per Day*	
	Boys	*Girls*
1	900-1200	800-1200
2	1100-1300	1000-1250
3	1100-1400	1050-1350
4	1200-1500	1150-1450
5	1300-1600	1200-1500
6	1500-1900	1450-1800
7	1600-2100	1500-1900
8	1700-2300	1600-2200
9	1900-2500	1800-2500
10	2100-2700	1900-2600
11	2100-2800	2000-2800
12	2300-3000	2100-3000
13	2500-3500	2300-3400
14	2600-3800	2400-3000
15	2700-4000	2400-2800
16	2700-4000	2250-2800
17	2800-4000	2250-2800

The late Dr. Mary S. Rose developed a system of *dietary distribution standards* for children which employs the principle of indicating what percentage of the total calories is to come from each chief kind or type of food. Table 13.3. shows such standards for children from 4 to 12 years of age, arranged in five age groups.

Table 13.3. Distributions of Calories in Diets of Children of 4 to 12 Years

Age	*Per cent of total Calories from each Class of Food*					
Years	*Foods from Cereal Grains*	*Milk*	*Vegetables and Fruits*	*Fats a*	*Sugars and Sweets*	*Eggs, Cheese, Meat and Other Flesh Foods*
4-5	23-25	45-50	14-18	5-8	2-5	5-6
5-6	23-25	45-50	14-18	5-8	2-5	5-6
6-7	20-25	40-45	14-15	10-12	3-4	4-5
8-9	20-25	38-42	15-16	12-13	4-6	5-8
10-12	20-25	34-38	17-18	13-14	6-8	7-8

In Table 13.4 are listed the minimum cost stands and moderate cost standards for children of ages 5 to 16 years.

Table 13.4. Distribution of Calories in Diets of Minimum and of Moderate Cost for Children of Ages 5 to 16 Years

Food Group	*Minimum Cost Diet Per Cent of Total Calories*	*Moderate Cost Diet Per cent of Total Calories*
I. Foods from cereal grains	37	24
II. Milk	22	32
III. Vegetables and fruits		
A. Dried legumes	3	1
B. Other vegetables and fruits	13	16
IV. Fats and oils	14	12
V. Sugars and sweets	5	7
VI. Meat, eggs, cheese	6	8

The Principle of Natural and Nutritional Wholes

An organism is more than a mere summation of its part, it is an *organized whole* and functions as such in nature. Many of nature's wholes have evolved under the influence of each other which have been more or less fixed by evolutionary process.

It is doubtless true that if we tried to subsist upon mixture of the known chemical essentials in artificially purified forms we might sooner or later find ourselves inadequately nourished for lack of something still unknown. Yet it is also true that if instead of artificially purified foodstuffs we use natural foods such as have constituted a part of the environment in which our bodies have evolved and to which they are nutritionally adjusted, then any essentials which may be still unknown are consumed as they occur in the natural wholes which we eat.

Closely related to the principle of natural wholes is that of nutritional flexibility.

The Principle of Nutritional Flexibility

It has already been stated that the body not only an organized natural whole but is something more than a mere summation. It is also *as organism* and so it is much more than a machine.

We may call the metabolic process "mechanistic" only in the sense that we formulate our concepts of it in physico-chemical terms which do not depend upon the assumption of any wholly mysterious vitalism. Yet, this concept should incorporate the fact that the body possesses an important degree of flexibility in its nutritional processes.

Due to this the body can make nutritional adjustments, and thus we can make good use of somewhat fluctuating food supplies.

This principle of nutritional flexibility is only in part a matter of simply raising or lowering the level of metabolism of a given factor, though at times this may be very important. There are also many cases of what is known sparing of one nutrient by another; and such cases are not all of any one chemical category. Three illustrations of nutritional flexibility given below:

(1) To some extent the body can adjust itself to a lowered total food intake by lowering its rate of basal energy metabolism, as also a loss of weight that reduces their expenditure of energy involved in bodily activities, external and internal. Benedict found that healthy young men could reduce their daily food calories by about one-third, partly by loss of weight and partly by lowered

basal metabolism. And in these cases the subjects continued their accustomed mental work and physical exercise and experienced little adverse effect beyond a diminution of animal spirits. Under severe wartime food restrictions, there have appeared to be much more drastic reductions of energy metabolism; but how far these have been physiological adjustments and how far pathological is not definitely known.

(2) By liberal intakes of carbohydrates and fats in order to make exceptional use of their protein-sparing powers, the rate of protein metabolism can be reduced to 30 grams a day or less in healthy, normally active men. This fact has been familiar for so long that its significance as an example of flexibility in nutrition is perhaps commonly overlooked.

(3) A recent example among vitamin is the finding that riboflavin can in some sense "spare" thiamine as shown by the fact that rats from families on high riboflavin diet show increased ability to endure shortage of thiamine.

These three examples are chemically so different as to indicate that the general principle of nutritional flexibility is of wide application.

With the help of feeding or injection experiments with nutrients (or compounds of nutritionally essential elements) containing "tagged" atoms, it has been possible to show that nutrient material received by the body is distributed promptly and widely to the various organs and tissues where it may be transformed in either one way or another. Flexibility is thus a more important aspect of nutrition than previously appreciated. But as was pointed out as early as 1939, is the fact that the isotopes of an element are not quite identical in chemical properties, and this is especially true of the elements of relatively low atomic weight which in general include those chiefly concerned in nutritional processes. Hence, the indications available from biochemical experiments with isotopic tracers should be investigated further by long-term feeding experiments with natural foodstuffs.

This nutritional flexibility means, that with a careful, continuing translation of our laboratory findings into terms of food commodities it is possible now to use our total food resources, or a so-called surplus of any of them, in such flexible but scientifically guided ways as to make them function more effectively for widespread nutritional well-being than we formerly knew how.

Harmonizing the Criteria of Dietary Adequacy and Nutritional Status

There is no denying the fact that the actual prevalence of malnutrition is much greater than is indicated by statistics of morbidity and mortality, or by hospital records. The reasons that so much of the malnutrition goes unrecognized are several: The more delicate methods for the diagnosis of the different nutritional deficiencies have been developed only so recently that relatively few physicians have the advanced knowledge and equipment required to make comprehensive, up-to-date examinations in this field of medicine; so the larger number of cases of malnutrition are not seen by anyone in position to recognize them and are reported according to such symptoms as point to some more commonly recognized disease. And also there are traditional priorities in the classifications of patients and of causes of deaths, so that even when the attending physician does report a nutritional deficiency the supervisory hospital official or the registrar of deaths will still probably classify the illness or death is essentially case of some disease more commonly recognized than are most types of malnutrition.

However, when the kinds and amounts of foods consumed by a fair sample of families are computed to their nutrient values and compared with the National Research Councils's Recommended Allowances, an appreciable proportion of these dietaries fall short of this standard in respect to one or more of their nutrient values. Some critics have held that either the dietary observations must be at fault or the Recommended Allowances must constitute too high a standard by which to judge adequacy, inasmuch as practicing physicians do not find nearly so many cases of malnutrition as the dietary studies would seem to imply.

It is true that the Recommended Allowances aim at adequacy for *best results* and not merely for prevention of disease. Also, in the use of such an eight-or nine-point "yardstick" there is an increased chance that an accidental fluctuation in the food supply might make an apparent shortage at some one point which in practice might be fully compensated with in the next few days.

Hence we should be careful to distinguish between the nutritional adequacy of the dietary, on the one hand, and the nutritional status of the body on the other.

If, the best methods of study are used there is reasonable harmony between the findings of dietary studies and the surveys of nutritional status, it is well for use also to realize that the two modes of enquiry do not measure quite the same thing, and that precise parallelism is not to be expected. In general, it is to be expected that an increase or decrease of nutrient intake will influence the level of concentration of the nutrient in the body's tissues and fluids more quickly than it will influence the structural tissue changes seen in biomicroscopy.

Thus there may not be complete and precise accord even as between the more chemical and the more physical of the delicate diagnostic methods. But neither as between these two types of methods of studying bodily status, nor as between either of them and a careful dietary survey, is there occasion for serious lack of confidence in the essential significance of the new knowledge.

14

Nutrition Needs of Children

14.1. Introduction

So far we have been considering the various nutrients in foods and their functions in the animal body. In this paper an attempt will be made to know in detail the nutritional requirements of children. It should be clearly understood that the nutritional life really does not begin with birth but it begins during the prenatal period and is influenced even earlier. The well-being of the infant is influenced not only by the diet of the mother during pregnancy but also by her status of nutrition prior to that period. A mother who is poorly nourished tends to give her baby a poor start in life nutritionally.

14.2. Needs During First Year

If we give proper attention to the kind, amount and sanitation of food as also the manner of feeding the baby will be a healthy and happy baby. During this period the nutrient requirements are high per unit of body weight because of rapid growth and since no reserves are available so the child must rely on his daily food supply for all his requirements of various nutrients.

After birth the child progressively accumulates subcutaneous fat for about nine months, after which the amount diminishes. However, by one year be becomes healthy and slender. If the muscle tissue of an infant feel firm, it shows a good nutritional status of the child. The growth of the child is quite rapid during first-nine months after birth Approx 2lb a month may be added to his body weight during first three months and then about 1lb a month. Similar pattern is noticed in respect of his height, there is an increase of about 20% in first three months and then it slows down and by one year the total increase is about 50% of the length (height) at birth.

Breast Feeding v/s Artificial Feeding

The most common food for a human infant is human milk. However, during recent times there has been a trend towards less breast feeding. In America more women of the "upper" economic educational class breast feed their infants than women of middle class. In India fewer women of higher socio - economic class breast feed their infants than women of middle class. The Indian trend is observed in other developing countries of the world.

Though we may improve the artificial feeds provided to the infants to such a level that there may not be any nutritional advantage in prescribing human milk for them. However, there shall still be certain advantages of breast feeding. Some of these are

- *(i)* Mother's milk (breast feeding) is free from bacterial contamination.
- *(ii)* It requires no preparation.
- *(iii)* It has lesser chances to be associated with infant eczema and other allergies.
- *(iv)* It is most economical.

Whether or not breast feeding improves parent - child relationship is controversial. It has been indicated by recent studies that "warmth and nervous stability of the mother" are more important than whether the child is breast fed or fed by bottle.

How to Supply the Required Nutrients

Since milk is the most common food and the composition of milk varies from species to species. We will restrict ourselves to human and cow milk which are generally given to infants though goats, milk is also fed to infants in some cases.

If we make a comparison between cow's milk and mother's milk, we find that human milk contains more lactose, iron, ascorbic acid and vitamin A per unit of volume. However, it contains less of protein, calcium phosphorus, riboflavin and thiamine.

The various nutrients present in milk will now be discussed in brief.

Carbohydrates: Lactose is the carbohydrate in all milks. In cow's milk its quantity is about $\frac{2}{3}$rd as to that found in human milk.

In artificial feeds some form of carbohydrate is added. Commonly used are sucrose and corn sirup. These sugars taste sweet and that is the only disadvantage associated with them Lactose (carbohydrate in natural milk) is the least tasting of all common sugars. In artificial feed lactose is not used because it is expensive combinations of maltose and dextrin which taste less sweet than sugar and sirup have been successfully used in infant formulas.

A comparison between the mother's milk and the cow's milk is shown in figures 14.1 and 14.2:

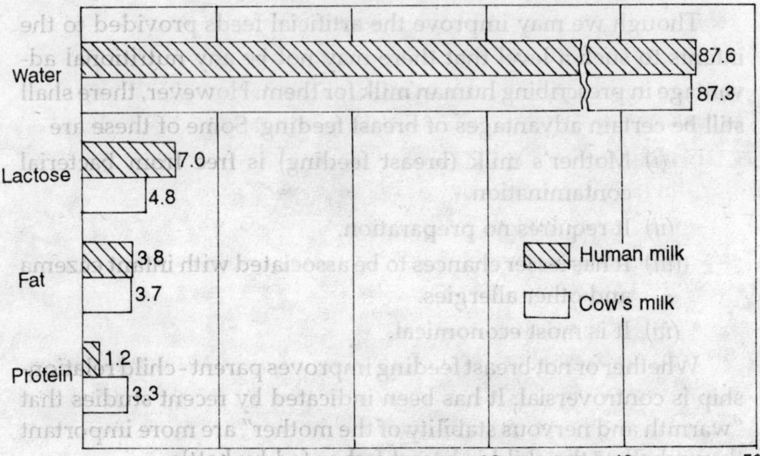

Fig.14.1. Composition of human and cows' milk in grams of water, lactose, fat and protein in 100 ml of milk.

Protein: We find the protein content of cow's milk to be three times to that of the mother's milk. Casein content of cow's milk is also higher as compared to human milk but the lactalhumin content of cow's milk is lower in comparison to human milk.

If the infant is fed with Raw cow's milk then it forms large, firm curds in his stomach but if diluted with water softer curds are formed. Similarly softer curds are formed when the cow's milk is given a heat treatment, acidification and homogenization.

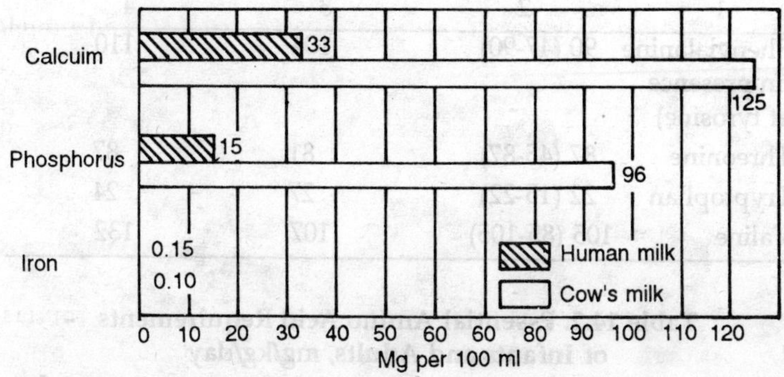

Fig.14.2. Calcium, phosphorus, and iron content of human and cow's milk.

From various studies carried out it has been clearly established that the amino acid needs of the infants and those of adults are quite different. Infants need then for growth and the adults for their nitrogen equilibrium. The need of infants is much greater than on the basis of their body weight unit as compared to adults.

These comparisons are listed in Tables 14.1 and 14.2 respectively.

Table 14.1. Essential Amino Acid Requirements of Infants Compared with Intake in Human Milk and Cow's Milk

Amino Acid	*Minimum Requirement (mg/kgday)*	*Human Milk (150ml/kg/day)*	*Cows' Milk (2.0 gm Protein per kg per day)*
1	2	3	4
Histidine	34 (16-34)	35	45
Isoleucine	126 (80-126)	102	122
Leucine	150 (76-229)	162	216
Lysine	103 (88-103)	114	156
Methionine (in presence of cystine)	45 (33-45)	50	58

(contd.)

1	2	3	4
Phenylalanine (in presence of tyrosine)	90 (47-90)	104	110
Threonine	87 (45-87)	81	87
Tryptophan	22 (15-22)	27	24
Valine	105 (85-105)	107	132

Table 14.2. Essential Amino Acid Requirements of Infants and Adults, mg/kg/day

Amino Acid	*Infant Requirement*	*Adult Requirement*		
		Men	*Women*	*Average*
Histidine	34	—	—	—
Isoleucine	126	10.4	5.2	7.8
Leucine	150	9.9	7.1	8.5
Lysine	103	8.8	3.3	6.1
Methionine (in presence of cystine)	45	—	3.9	3.9
phenylalanine (in presence of tyrosine)	90	4.3	3.1	3.7
Threonine	87	6.5	3.5	5.0
Tryptophan	22	2.9	2.1	2.5
Valine	105	8.8	9.1	9.0

The NRC recommended a daily protein intake of the infant upto one year at 2.5 ± 0.5 g per kg of body weight. The allowance per kg decrease progressively from birth. Breast feeding provides the infant an intake of about 1.5 to 2.0g of protein per kg of body weight during the first six months of life.

Fat: There is not much appreciable difference in the fat content of human milk and cow's milk as both contain about 3.5-4.0 g of fat per 100 ml of milk. they however differ in their fatty acid contents. The proportion of saturated fatty acids is more in cow's milk where as mother's milk is found to contain more of unsaturated fatty acids. The fatty acid content is listed in Table 14.3.

Table 14.3. Distribution of Some of the Lipid Components in Human and Cow's Milk

	gm/100gm Milk Fat Mature Milk	
	Human	*Cow*
Total fat	3.8	3.7
Fatty acid distribution		
Saturated fatty acids		
Butyric	0.4	3.1
Caproic	0.1	1.0
Caprylic	0.3	1.2
Capric	1.7	2.6
Unsaturated fatty acids		
Linoleic (octadecadienoic)	8.3	1.6
Arachidonic	0.8	1.0

Minerals: The amount of calcium in cow's milk is three times of that found in human milk per unit volume. A breast fed infant gets about 60mg calcium per kg body weight but if fed on cow's milk he gets about 160 mg calcium per kg of the body weight. The % age of calcuim retained is higher for human milk (66 %) than for cows' milk (35-50%). The breast fed babies get enough of calcium. The recommended allowance of calcium is 0.7g daily for artificially fed infant during first year of life.

Iron: Only a little of iron is found to be present in both (i.e. cow's milk and human milk). From a study done on pregnant women by transfusion of blood containing radio active irons we have been able to find the capacity of the infant to retain fetal iron. At the birth an infant contains 80 mg iron per kg of body weight, out of it about 50 mg/kg is in blood, 25 mg/kg is present as storage iron (divided equally between liver and other tissues) and 5 mg/kg is found in bone marrow, myoglobin and intracellular enzymes.

The infant is thus born with a store of iron that body holds tenaciously, using it through out infancy.

At birth the hemoglobin level is 22 g/100 ml (high) which comes down to about 10.5 - 11.5 g/100 ml at about three months of age. At this age the child may be provided with iron rich foods such as egg yolk, green vegetables, meats and enriched cereals.

In developing countries we came across cases of iron deficiency anemia in infants. It has been found that fortification of a prepared milk formula with iron 12 mg per quart is sufficient to maintain hemoglobin and serum iron concentrations at normal levels.

The fact that the source of fetal iron is maternal plasma is supported by following study, which was carried out on rabbit using radioactive iron. It was observed as the pregnancy progressed, relatively less of plasma iron entered the maternal bone marrow and more was directed to the fetus. Near the end of the prenatal period the fetus was getting around 90% of the total iron carried in the maternal plasma.

NRC recommended allowance for iron is 1.0 mg/kg of body for infants from 3 to 12 months.

The Vitamins

Vitamin A: The total vitamin A in milk is the sum of performed vitamin A and the cartinoid pigments.

In human milk the proportion of carotinoid vitamin is lesser than that of performed vitamin A where as in cow's milk their proportions are approximately same.

NRC recommended 1500 IU of vitamin A daily for infants through out first year of their life. This much of vitamin A is present in about 1 quart of cow's milk.

Vitamin content of milk are listed in Table 14.4

Table 14.4. Vitamin Content of Human and Cows' Milk

(per 100 ml Whole Milk)

Vitamin	*Human*	*Cow*
A, μg	53	34
Carotenoids, μg	27	38
D, IU	0.42	2.36
Ascorbic acid, mg	4.3	1.6
Niacin, μg	172	85
Riboflavin, μg	42.6	157
Thiamine, μ	16	42

Thiamine

NRC recommended allowance for thiamine is 0.4 mg/day upto one year of age. The average thiamine content of human milk is 0.21 mg/100 Calories and from any milk formula we do not get more than 0.24 mg/1000 Cal. Thus the diet should be supplemented to provide for thiamine during the first year of life. For this the diet should include enriched cereals eggs, meat and vegetables.

Riboflavin

The riboflavin content of cow's milk depends upon the breed of the cow and in mother's milk it depends upon the diet of the mother and its average concentration is 0.6 mg/ 1000 Cal. which is about 3 to 4 times of that in cow's milk.

The recommended daily allowance for riboflavin infants is 0.6 mg during first year.

Niacin

The amount of niacin is approximately double in human milk as compared to cow's milk. In human milk it is about 7.5 mg/1000 Calories.

The recommended daily allowance of niacin is 0.60 mg equivalent per 1000 calories.

Ascorbic Acid

The ascorbic acid content of human milk is found to depend on the diet of the mother but it is more in comparison to that of the cow's milk. For safety it is usually recommended for the breast fed as also bottle fed infants. Orange juice is the most common source.

The recommended allowance for it is 30 mg daily during first year. This much amount is available in about $\frac{1}{4}$th cup of orange juice.

Vitamin D: The amount of vitamin D in human milk depends upon mother's diet. However, a supplemental source of vitamin D is recommended for both, breast fed and bottle fed infants. The recommended allowance of vitamin D is 135 IU to prevent rickets. However a better growth occurs with 300 - 400 IU daily and so the recommend allowance in 400 IU daily.

Solid Foods

It is generally recommended that the babies should be given some solid food by the time they are 5-6 months or age. They are particularly needed to supply iron and thiamine but they make valuable contribution to the intake of other nutrients as well.

To start with enriched cereals are added and then pureed fruit. The pureed vegetables them become a part of the diet. Egg yolks and strained meat are also added to diet.

THE PRE - SCHOOL CHILDREN
(During Years 2-6)

The pre-school child grows relatively more in height and takes an appearance of being taller and thinner. The well nourished per-school child is sturdily built and becomes more like an adult in posture and stride. His nutritional needs depend upon his growth, activity, status of nutrition etc. In general following Principles may be applied.

Energy: The suggested energy requirements are

1—3 years	1300 Cal
3—6 years	1600 Cal

For further details see Table 14.5.

Ideal supplements to increase the calorie intake are foods rich in nutrient content such as milk,. fruits, vegetables and cereals (whole grain or enriched). It is desirable to avoid concentrated sweets and foods high in fat.

Protein: The recommended daily allowance is 32g for 1-3 years, 40g for 3-6 years, of age. It provides approximately 10% of calories needed.

Foods that provide protein to children of this age group are milk (a glass at each meal will provide 20-24g daily), an egg (6g).

Calcium: The recommended daily allowance is 0.8g during the 1-9 years of age.

Table 14.5. Recommended Daily Dietary Allowances. Designed for the Maintenance of good Nutrition

	Age[1], Years	Weight *kg*	Weight *(lb)*	Height *cm*	Height *(in.)*	*Energy, Cal.*	*Protein, gm*	*Calcium, gm*	*Iron, mg*	*Vitamin A Value, IU*	*Thiamine, mg*	*Riboflavin, mg*	*Niacin Equiv. mg*	*Ascorbic Acid mg*	*Vitamin D, IU*
Children	1-3	13	(29)	87	(34)	1300	32	0.8	8	2000	0.5	0.8	9	40	400
	3-6	18	(40)	107	(42)	1600	40	0.8	10	2500	0.6	1.0	11	50	400
	6-9	24	(53)	124	(49)	2100	52	0.8	12	3500	0.8	1.3	14	60	400
Boys	9-12	33	(72)	140	(55)	2400	60	1.1	15	4500	1.0	1.4	16	70	400
	12-15	45	(98)	156	(61)	3000	75	1.4	15	5000	1.2	1.8	20	80	400
	15-18	61	(134)	172	(68)	3400	85	1.4	15	5000	1.4	2.0	22	80	400
Girls	9-12	33	(72)	140	(55)	2200	55	1.1	15	4500	0.9	1.3	15	80	400
	12-15	47	(103)	158	(62)	2500	62	1.3	15	5000	1.0	1.5	17	80	400
	15-18	53	(117)	163	(64)	2300	58	1.3	15	5000	0.9	1.3	15	70	400

Iron: The recommended daily allowance is 8.0 mg for 1-3 years of age and 10mg for 3-6 years of age. However, it is not easy to supply this much irons unless some iron-enriched foods are included in daily diet. Eggs, meat, green vegetable etc. can provide 1mg of iron to child. Enriched and whole grain bread supply about 0.5 mg per slice, enriched cereals supply 0.5 - 1 mg per serving. One and a half point milk supply 0.3 mg of iron. Most of the fruits provide less than 0.5 mg per serving.

Table 14.6. Iron Requirement of Children

	5 Years of Age		*10 years of Age*	
Function	*Boys mg/day*	*Girls mg/day*	*Boys mg/day*	*Girls mg/day*
Growth	0.2	0.3	0.4	0.5
Maintenance	0.3	0.3	0.4	0.4
Storage	0.1	0.1	0.2	0.4
Total to absorb	0.6	0.7	1.0	1.3
Food-iron required	6.0	7.0	7.0	9.0
National Research Council Allowance	8.0	8.0	12.0	12.0

A general pattern of foods for a good daily diet for the pre-school child is given in Table 14.6.

Table 14.7. Food for the Day for the Pre-school Child

Food	*Amounts*	*Comments*
1	2	3
Milk	**2 to 3 cups**	Some children do not have this capacity at the pre-school age. If your child does not, let him drink what he wants and try to get in more by using it in cooking.
Meat or fish or poultry	**1 serving**	Beef, lamb, pork, poultry, fish or liver may be used. Occasionally cheese may be substituted for a serving of meat. (For an average serving at this age, nutritionists sometimes estimate about one level tablespoon of meat or vegetables per year of age. But this is no hard and fast rule. In serving food to a young child, put on his plate only what you think he will eat).

(contd.)

1	2	3		
Egg	1			
Potatoes	1 average serving			
Vegetables	1 or 2 average servings of green or yellow	Suggestions:		
		Carrots	Cabbage	Lettuce
		Spinach	Squash	Green peas
		Green beans	Broccoli	Green peppers
		Tomatoes	Celery	
Fruits	2 average servings	One of these to be orange or grapefruit for vitamin C		
Cereal	1 average serving	Whole-grain or enriched		
Bread	3 slices	Whole-grain or enriched		
Butter or fortified margarine	2 tbsp			
Vitamin D supplement	As recommended by physician			

Nutritional Requirements

The nutritional requirements of a child depend upon his rate of growth. The nutrient is needed also for energy, regulating body temperature, repair of tissues etc.

In the years 7-13 years of age the growths continues at a steady pace. In boys the growth spurt begins around 13-15 years of age and in girls around 10-11 years of age and they continue to grow rapidly for 4-5 years during the adolescent period. The rate of growth then tapers off to the relatively small gains of characteristics of adulthood as final body size in approached.

During the age of 7-18 years the daily nutrient requirements increase with each advance in age for boys and to the age 15 years for girls. The nutrient requirements of teenagers (boys) is highest in their life time. In case of girls the teenager girls have higher requirement than at any earlier time but less than those for women during pregnancy and lactation. The needs of adolescent are influenced greatly by their rapid growth. The recommendation given in Table 14.5 is useful when applied to groups of children but due to wide variation in body size and rate of growth during the adolescence it may penalize some children by being too limited and may prove too generous for others.

The recommended allowances for boys 12 to 15 years of age is 3000 Cal. daily; and to take care of the continuing rapid rate of growth in the 15 to 18 year period, 3400 Cal. For girls, 12 to 15 years, 2500 Cal. are recommended; with growth tapering off in the 15 to 18 year period the allowance is decreased to 2300 Cal.

It is not so easy to assess the adequacy of the protein, mineral, and vitamin intake as it is energy. Three extensive series of studies have contributed to the knowledge of nutritional needs and status of children. Macy and her coworkers in Detroit observed children 4 to 12 years of age, measuring the intake and excretion of eighteen chemical substances. In a Southern regional experiment station project, the needs of the preadolescent girls were investigated for energy, protein, calcium, iron, phosphorus, magnesium, cobalt, copper, manganese, molybdenum, zinc, sulfur, vitamin A, carotene, riboflavin, folic acid, vitamin B_{12}, and pantothenic acid. At the Washington Agricultural Experiment Station the nutritional status of adolescent children and the dietary intake of vitamin A, ascorbic acid, riboflavin, and niacin were determined. These series of studies and other research are reflected in the Recommended daily allowances for children (Table 14.5.).

Values for the minimum requirement for eight essential amino acids have been suggested by Nakagawa and his coworkers of Tokyo for preadolescent boys. The investigators patterned the amino acid mixture used and the procedure followed after that of Rose. In brief, a negative nitrogen balance is induced by withdrawal of an essential amino acid from the mixture. On replacement of the amino acid, the least amount required to maintain a positive nitrogen balance is considered the minimal need. Removal of neither arginine nor histidine induced a negative balance. With seven of the amino acids, all except tryptophan, the estimated minimal amino acid requirement for the boys, on the basis of total for the day, exceeded that for the adults. Amino acid needs have been investigated quantitatively only relatively recently. Further study of more persons may of course bring some changes in values. The sample meals for adolescent are given below:-

A Sample Day's Meals for A 10-Year-Old

Breakfast

Tomato juice (3/4 c)
Hot whole wheat cereal (2/3 c) with milk (1/2 c)
Toast (2 sl)with butter or fortified margarine (2 tsp)
Milk (1/2 pt)

Lunch

(If served at school or at home)
Creamed eggs (3/4 c)
Green beans (1/2 c) with butter or fortified margarine (1 tsp)
Oatmeal muffins (2) with butter or fortified margarine (1 tsp)
Milk (1/2 pt)
(If brought from home)
Sandwich-peanut butter and raw carrot on buttered whole-grain or enriched bread
Supplemented at school by—
Orange
Milk soup (1 c) or cocoa (1 c)
Sandwich-chopped dried fruit buttered whole-grain or enriched bread
Supplemented at school by—
Orange
Milk soup (1 c) or cocoa (1 c)

Dinner

Meat loaf (1 serving)
Scalloped potatoes (2/3 c)

Coleslaw with red and green peppers (1/2 c)

Whole wheat bread or enriched bread (2 sl) with butter or fortified margarine (2 tbsp)

applesauce (1/2 c)

Molasses cookies (2 thin)

Milk (1/2 pt)

Snacks of fruit, milk, Graham crackers.

A Sample Day's Meals for an Adolescent Boy

Breakfast

Orange (1 med)

Shredded wheat with milk (1/2 c)

Eggs (2)

Muffins (3) with butter or fortified margarine (2 tbsp) and marmalade (2 tbsp) Cocoa (2 c).

Lunch

Macaroni and cheese (2 lg servings)

Sliced tomatoes (2) with mayonnaise (1 tbsp)

Rye bread (2 med sl) with butter or fortified margarine (1 tbsp)

Baked apple (1 lg) with sugar (1 tbsp) and cream (1/4 c)

Cookies (2 large)

Milk (1/2 pt).

Dinner

Pot roast of beef (lg serving)

Baked Potato with gravy

Cabbage (1 c) with butter or fortified margarine (2 tbsp)

Whole wheat bread (2 med sl) with butter or fortified margarine (1 tbsp)

Rice milk pudding (2 servings)

Milk (1/2 pt)

Snacks of fruit, milk, cookies, sandwiches.

15

Nutritional Chemistry of Reproduction and Lactation

15.1. Nutritional Needs of Pregnancy

There is no doubt in the fact that the function of gestation increases the nutrition need. To support it we take into consideration researches carried out at Harvard Medical School and in Torasto which have shown that both mother and child profit greatly by superior feeding during pregnancy. Mendenhall writes, "To count on the fact that the mother is a factor of safety in the nutrition of the young, and to nourish the child at the expense of the pragnant or nourishing mother is an unnecessary sacrifice of the woman and may at any time move disastrous to the child". And also "those is every reason to believe that ability to produce breast milk of a superior quality is to some extent dependent as the storage of material from the mother's food during the prenatal period, as well as on the supply of nutrients from the food the receives during lactation."

The increase in the energy metabolism becomes measurable after about four months of pregnancy and then rises steadily until at term it is about 25% greater than for the same woman during reproductive rest.

In submitting its recommendations of 1948 the National Research Council stated that "as to the most desirable levels of calorie intake during pregnancy and lactation, the allowances recommended.... seek a middle ground within the somewhat broad range of present professional opinion."

Hunscher, et al. (1935) found that with generous amounts of proteins in the diet, the maternal organism tended to store nitrogen greatly in excess of the amounts retained in the fetus and its adnexa; and that this maternal reserve acted to offset the strongly negative nitrogen balances of the subsequent (in the case which they studied, unusually heavy) lactation period.

However, Coons found that in pregnant woman who chose diet in which protein content was lower than usual (about 11g of nitrogen a day) and the retention of nitrogen were not in all cases as high as the amount presumably transferred to the fetus. He also found that low storage of nitrogen during pregnancy might adversely effect lactation.

The body of a normal infant at the five of birth is found to contain about 60g of nitrogen, 20g of calcium, 15g of phosphorus are contained is the body.

Macy and Hunscher have computed that under favourable nutritional conditions, the mother's positive balance during pregnancy is about 500g of nitrogen, 65g of phosphorous, 29g of calcium these figures indicate 700-800% more of nitrogen, 300-400% more of phosphorus, 25-50% more of calcium than is contained is the body of the baby at birth.

To an extent not yet clearly defined, these surpluses appear to represent the laying up by the mother during pregnancy of nutritional reserves against the heavy demands of lactation. Macy and coworkers (Hummel, et al., 1936) show by prolonged balance studies the practicability of providing through the food for such liberal storage of protein, calcium, magnesium and phosphorus.

The studies about iron have already been described in the previous Chapter 13.

In regions in which the environment provides no liberal margin of iodide intake (in general, the goiterous regions), iodine deficiency may be induced by the extra demands of pregnancy and lactation. Medical advice should be sought in safeguarding against this danger.

Vitamin requirements are undoubtedly increased in pregnancy, and we have no ground for assuming that the increase is the same or closely similar in the case of each vitamin. Abundance of vitamin A has been shown to be very beneficial.

15.2. Division of the Penalty of Malnutrition between the Mother and the Offspring

To great extent, the organism of the mother serves as a "factor of safety" in the nutrition of the young both before birth and during lactation. Sometimes, however, this important principle,- that Nature is "more careful" of the perpetuation of the race than of the conservation of the adult-may be overemphasized. Thus it is an exaggeration to say that the unborn offspring "is a perfect parasite upon the mother." It is in a sense a "parasite" but not a "perfect" one in the sense of taking just as much from the mother whether she has it spare or not.

The fetus may draw heavily upon the mother, taking material beyond that which the mother can well spare but when the nutritional intake is seriously deficient to the total demand of pregnancy it must be expected that both the mother and the young will be unfavourably affected.

This is illustrated in the experiment carried out upon young milch cattle at the University of Wisconsin. Four groups of young females were placed on four rations derived respectively from the wheat plant, the oat plant, the corn (maize) plant, and a mixture of the three. By mixing proper proportions of the leaves and stalk of the plant with its seed (and when necessary supplementing with some of a protein-concentrate of the same seed) all four rations were given the same energy and protein content. Growth was completed on all four of these rations; but the reproduction and lactation records were very different. Here, because pregnancy and lactation imposed such heavy nutritional demands, a diet which was satisfactory even for growth fell short of the needs for satisfactory bearing and suckling of young. Thus, support of reproduction and lactation becomes a delicate test of the quality of a diet.

15.3. Nutritional Support of Lactation in the Human Mother

Experimentation upon milk production has shown that not more than two third of the extra calories fed are recovered in the milk, or conversely, that the extra food requirement (in calories) is at least 50% greater than the number of extra calories in the milk produced. In the work of Shukers. Macy, el al. (1931) it was found that: "Lactation increases the food demands (of the human mother) approximately 60% over and above those of pregnancy." The actual voluntary food intakes found in two unusually successfully lactating women were 4600 and 4800 Calories per day, respectively.

In cases wherein the physician believes that liberal feeding of the mother may help in establishing the activity of promoting the productivity of her mammary glands, it is doubtless wise (at least until knowledge in this field becomes more precise) to make the dietary liberal in respect to all nutritional factors; for the consensus of competent opinion is clearly in favour of the nursing of the baby by the mother, in all reasonably normal cases. And physicians are increasingly successful in stimulating human milk secretion.

Yet it may also be said that something in human evolution or in the conditions of present-day civilizations seems to have worked at some cost of the natural function of human lactation, so that even with the best of nutrition the mother may not secrete as much milk as the baby needs. When the physician is thoroughly convinced that this is true of the individual case, the fact may be accepted without any undue feeling of defeat.

Liberal feeding for the support of lactation should begin early; for it can safely be inferred from the results of animal experimentation that the ability to sustain a good rate of milk production depends largely upon the nutritional condition induced and maintained by good feeding from the beginning of the lactation period.

16

Nutrition During Pregnancy, Lactation, Aging

16.1. Nutrition During Pregnancy

Meeting both fetel and maternal requirements and hence setting up nutrient allowances for pregnancy has, for the most part, been based on the suggested allowances for the non-pregnant woman with the super imposed additional requirements for pregnancy. The diet of a pregnant woman deserves special consideration to ascertain a good health for both, the mother and the child. The influence of nutritions begins prior to conception and continues through out the gestation period. Certain ill effects have been associated with maternal consumption of a diet poor in nutritional quality. Generally Toxemia in mother and prematurity in infant are associated with inadequate diet of the pregnant woman other ill effects are miscarriages, premature and still births, illness and death resulting from illness etc.

One of the most extensive studies of prenatal nutrition was conducted at Vanderbilt University and included 2338 women of the lower income bracket. It was observed that when the mother's energy intake was 1500 Cal. or less or the protein less than 50 gm daily, the incidence of obstetric and fatal complications increased. However, the investigators showed that the lessened dietary intake may have been due to the complications rather than the cause of them.

The results of a study in India of 150 pregnant women of low socioeconomic strata and 50 pregnant women of high economic strata show that the nutritional status of women during pregnancy and the condition of the offspring were not notably different for the two groups. The investigators pointed out that the women who were consuming a deficient diet during pregnancy had subsisted on this type of diet since birth, and that perhaps some physiological adaptation to conserve nutrients was in affect? The Harvard investigators found that mothers with diets of good quality not only suffered fewer complications during pregnancy but also had less difficulty during labour. Furthermore, the mother had better prospectus of being able to nurse her infant if her had been of good quality during pregnancy (Fig. 16.1). As for the infant, the Harvard group found a definite all over relationship between excellence of the mother's diet and superiority in the physical status of the newborn (Fig. 16.2).

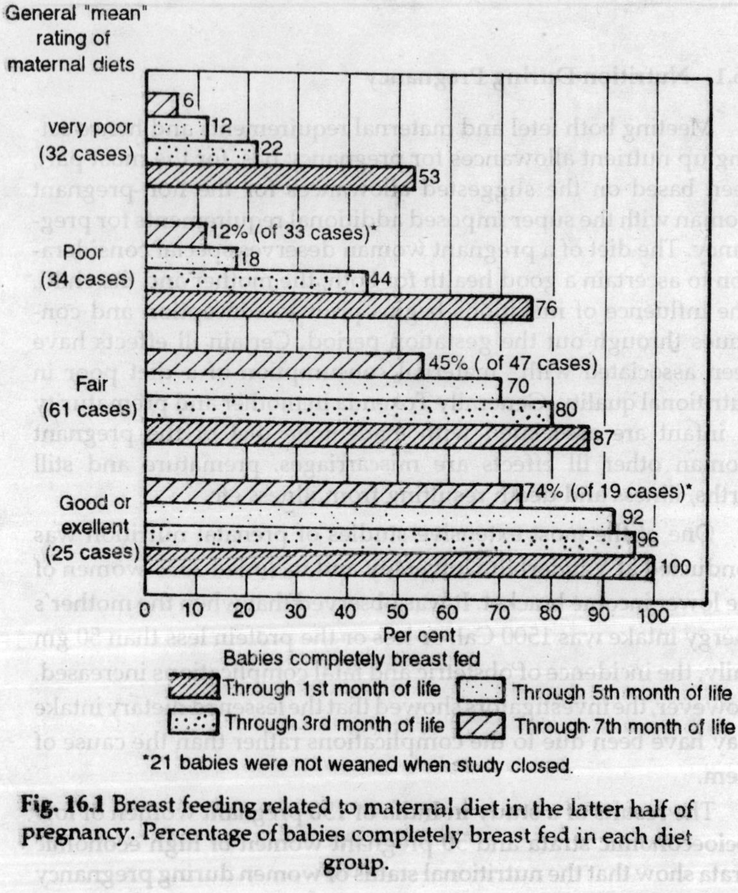

Fig. 16.1 Breast feeding related to maternal diet in the latter half of pregnancy. Percentage of babies completely breast fed in each diet group.

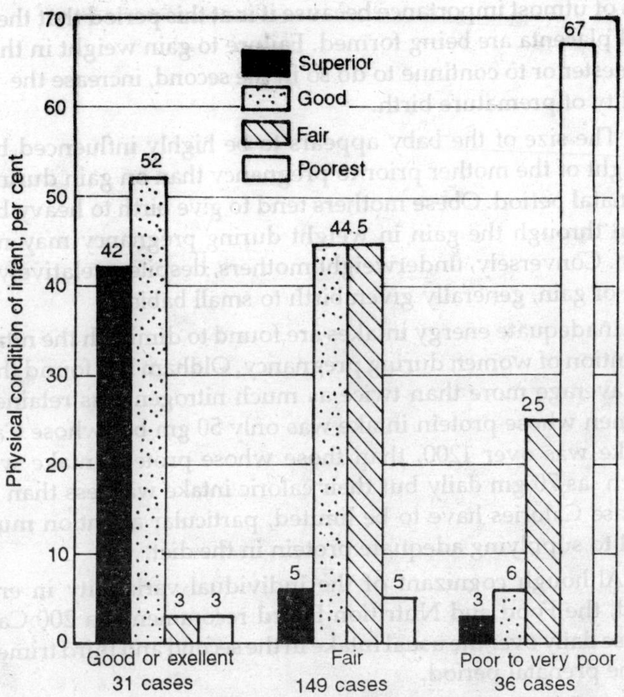

Fig. 16.2 Relationship of prenatal nutrition to the physical condition of the infant at birth and within first 2 weeks of life.

During the first eight weeks of the prenatal period the fetal organs are being formed. The second half is important since the majore gain in weight of the fetus occur during that period. Because of this the demands for building materials for the formation of new tissue get stepped up markedly. The maternal diet should provide for the additional needs. It should be recognized also that not only is the fetal tissue increasing in amount but also the mother too is experiencing a growth of certain tissues; the mammary glands, and accessory tissues supporting the fetus, as well as certain other glands and tissues throughout the body increase in size during the prenatal period.

Energy

Calorie intake is of special interest during pregnancy as it has a relationship to material weight gain. The pattern of gain and amount are significant to the well-being of the mother. During the first trimester, although the absolute increase in weight is small, it is of utmost importance because it is at this period that the fetus and placenta are being formed. Failure to gain weight in the first trimester or to continue to do so in the second, increase the probability of premature birth.

The size of the baby appears to be highly influenced by the weight of the mother prior to pregnancy than on gain during the prenatal period. Obese mothers tend to give birth to heavy babies even through the gain in weight during pregnancy may not be high. Conversely, underweight mothers, despite a relatively high rate of gain, generally given birth to small babies.

Inadequate energy intakes are found to diminish the nitrogen retention of women during pregnancy. Oldham has found that on the average more than twice as much nitrogen was retained by women whose protein intake was only 50 gm but whose Calorie intake was over 1200, than those whose protein intake was as much as 70 gm daily but their caloric intake was less than 2100. In case Calories have to be limited, particular attention must be paid to supplying adequate protein in the diet.

Although cognizant of the individual variability in energy need, the Food and Nutrition Board recommends a 200 Cal. increase daily over the usual intake in the second and third trimesters of the prenatal period.

Protein

The quantity of protein required during pregnancy is much more increased, special in the second half of pregnancy. Most of the protein acquisition by the fetus in the three months prior to birth. The rate of protein deposition in the fetus, computed for the entire prenatal period, is around 1.4 gm per day. For the last three months of fetal life the rate is increased to 3.6 gm daily, and for the last month the increase reaches an average of 6.4 gm daily. Added to this are the needs of the mother, which are increased to take care of the enlargement of certain of her own body tissues during the prenatal period. For the mother who is in a state of good nutrition prior to pregnancy and whose protein intake during the early months of the prenatal period has been at least at the recommended level, the Food and Nutrition Board recommends and additional 20 gm protein daily during the second and third trimesters.

The quantitative requirement for protein has been studied by means of the nitrogen balance method. From observations during the entire prenatal period, indications are that the body stores nitrogen to a greater extent than can be accounted for by the combined growth of the fetus and maternal tissues. Of course-there are additional demands for nitrogen, for at birth nitrogen is lost from the body in fluids and tissue in addition to the fetus, and during lactation the nitrogen balance is generally negative.

It has been concluded, that during pregnancy proteins of good quality should be eaten. Comparisons of the average excretions of amino acids by women in the pregnant and nonpregnant state show an increase in amino acid needs during pregnancy. In a study of the eight indispensable amino acids, the magnitude of increase varied among them. The greatest average increases were for theonine and tryptophan, followed by lysine. An increase in excretion is interpreted as evidence of a greater need for amino acid by the body.

Calcium

Factors that influence the calcium requirements during pregnancy are quite similar to those of protein. The amount needed is influenced by the growth both of fetal and maternal tissues, with the greatest need coming in the last prenatal month. At birth the fetus contains approximately 22 gm of calcium, most of which is deposited in the last fetal month. The rate of accumulation of calcium in the fetus is about 50 mg per day at the third month; 120 mg daily by the seventh, and by the last month it reaches 450 mg per day.

Daily dietary requirements for calcium have been determined by means of balance studies. For women in a state of good nutrition prior to the prenatal period, the Recommended Allowance for the second and third trimesters is an additional 0.5 gm per day more than the recommendation for a nonpregnant woman, amounting to a total 1.3 gm. Like protein, calcium is retained during pregnancy beyond the needs estimated for the fetal and new maternal tissues. Such storage is not amiss, for during lactation the diet frequently supplies an insufficient amount of calcium to meet the augmented requirement.

In cases of undernutrition prior to the prenatal period, the intake of calcium, protein, and other nutrients should be increased at the outset and continued throughout. Women with histories of poor nutrition prior to pregnancy, when given an adequate diet, are found to store more calcium than women on the same diet who entered pregnancy in a good nutritional state.

Iron

The recommended intake for iron during the second and third trimesters of the prenatal period is 20 mg daily. Like the other nutrients, the quantitative need increases with the progress of pregnancy.

It is only by careful selection of foods that 20 mg of iron can be provided in the daily diet. Thus it becomes necessary to be on the watch to include iron-rich foods. Foods that are good sources of iron are liver, other meats, eggs, enriched or whole-grain cereals and breads, green and leafy vegetables, and some dried fruits.

Hypochromic anemia is common in pregnancy. The previous lifetime iron balance is of importance in determining the iron reserve and the capacity to meet the demands of pregnancy. Some believe it to be only a manifestation of hydremia (excess of water in the blood). It can be prevented to a large extent by the ingestion of an adequate diet, although in some in some instances medicinal supplementation is desirable. There as two physiological changes that help compensate for the added demands for iron. During the period of gestation the cessation of menstruation represents a saving of iron amounting to 200 to 300 mg. Also it has been demonstrated, using radioactive iron, that iron absorption is increased during pregnancy, specially during the last trimester.

Iodine

During pregnancy the requirement for iodine gets increased. In Switzerland, where a serious lack of iodine exists in the soil, it has been observed that if mothers develop goiter because of an insufficient consumption of iodine, the possibilities of her child's also having goiter are ten times more.

In regions where the incidence of goiter was highest among the mothers cretinism was more apt to take place among the children. Where 55% of the people in a village were afflicted with endemic goiter, the incidence of cretinism was around 1%.

Under normal conditions the use of iodized salt may be sufficient to provide an adequate amount of iodine. However, with the increased need of pregnancy and the possibility of the intake of salt being restricted to medical reasons, it would seem wise to consult a physician concerning additional iodine intake. Such a practice is recommended particularly for persons living in areas where a lack of iodine is prevalent.

The Vitamins

The vitamin requirements during pregnancy have been less thoroughly studied than the protein and mineral requirements. It is logical to assume that there is an increased demand for these nutrients during the prenatal period. Research that has been done supports this point of view. The recommendations of the Food and Nutrition Board for the daily allowances of the vitamins are greater than the recommendations for nonpregnant women.

Vitamin A and D: For vitamin A value the Recommended Allowance for the second and third trimesters of pregnancy is 6000 IU daily, based on the assumption that two-thirds of the total vitamin A activity of the diet is derived from carotene and related compounds, and one-third from the preformed vitamin. The 6000 IU allowance daily can be supplied easily by the combination of one quart of milk, butter or fortified margarine, a green vegetable and occasionally liver.

Deprivation of vitamin A during pregnancy results certain physical abnormalities. Newborn rats and pigs were found to have cleft palates, defects of the skeletal structure and of the eyes. To the other extreme, excessive intake has also caused physical abnormalities in rats. Such extremes have not been recorded for the human being.

The optimum intake of vitamin D during pregnancy is not definitely known. The level suggested is 400 IU daily for the second and third trimesters of the prenatal period. The diet cannot be depended upon to supply this amount unless milk with added vitamin D is used. Readily available sources of the vitamin on the market include fish liver oils and irradiated sterols of many kinds and potencies. Clinical symptoms of vitamin D deficiency are rare in the United States and Europe. In India, China, and other areas of the Far East symptoms of osteomalacia (late rickets) do occur during reproduction. Among the women in the Far East who can appear in public only if veiled, the source of vitamin D from the sun is completely eliminated.

Ascorbic Acid: One hundred mg daily is the Recommended Allowanced for ascorbic acid during the second and third trimesters of pregnancy. Two servings of citrus fruit will supply the recommended intake. Tomatoes can be depended on to provide some of the vitamin; also cabbage, potatoes (under proper conditions of preparation), broccoli, strawberries, and cantaloup are among the good sources.

Evidence of an increased need for ascorbic acid is found in the study of maternal blood levels. As pregnancy progresses, the ascorbic acid concentration in the maternal blood tends to decrease. However, when the intake is maintained at a high level the customary progressive reduction does not occur.

Thiamine: The Recommended Allowance for thiamine for the second and third trimesters in 1 mg daily, which is slightly higher than the 0.4 mg per 1000 Cal. rate of the nonpregnant woman. Thiamine is supplied in good amounts by the following foods: whole-grain and enriched cereals containing approximately 0.8 mg per 1000 Cal.; whole milk, 0.5 mg per 1000 Cal.; and lean meats, an average of 0.3 mg per 1000 Cal.

The question of associating certain common symptoms manifested during pregnancy with an inadequate intake of thiamine arises periodically but remains controversial. Some investigators attribute the symptoms of general nervous fatigue, muscle cramps, neuritis, and toxemia to an insufficiency of thiamine; others disagree.

Riboflavin: The Recommended Allowance for riboflavin during the second and third trimesters is increased by 0.3 mg above the recommendation for women, making the daily allowance for pregnant women 18 to 35 years of age. 1.6 mg. The daily intake of one quart of milk, along with enriched bread and cereals, and the other foods in an average mixed diet, will supply the riboflavin allowance without difficulty.

In experimental studies with the rat, a lack of riboflavin specially at the thirteenth or fourteenth embryo day, may interfere with normal cartilage formation and result in malformations of the skeletal structure. Cleft palates and shortening of the mandible, tibia, fibula, radius, and toes were observed.

Vitamin E: Although it is well established that vitamin E (alpha tocopherol) is essential for reproduction in animals, the need for the human being is controversial. Some investigators have reported that vitamin E is beneficial for women who have had histories of repeated abortions whereas others have found it to be ineffective even though given in high dosages over long periods of time. Most agree that the levels of total tocopherols in the blood rise as gestation progresses.

Vitamin K: At one time it was common practice to administer vitamin K routinely during pregnancy and also to the newborn for the prevention of hemorrhage in the newborn child. The practice is now being questioned on the grounds that it is uncertain whether the decreased prothombin level characteristic of the newborn is a direct cause of hemorrhage. Furthermore, there is conflicting evidence as to whether or not vitamin K administration reduces the incidence of hemorrhage in the newborn. The more recent observations lend support to the belief that it is effective in reducing hemorrhage.

Foods Recommended in the Daily Diet

The following list of foods forms a basis for an adequate diet during pregnancy. However, variations may individual cases may be recommended by physicians.

Milk—3 or more cups of whole or skimmed milk.

Fruits and vegetables—5 to 7 servings of fruits and vegetables, including some green and leafy and some citrus fruits or tomatoes.

Lean meat, poultry, fish—at least one-quarter of a pound of meat or fish is desirable. It is well to include a serving of liver at intervals.

Eggs—at least one egg.

Cereals and bread—3 servings of enriched or whole-grained bread and cereals.

Butter and fortified margarine—should be used sparingly if weight is being watched.

Fluids and vitamin D are needed daily.

16.2. Nutrition During Lactation

During lactation the increase in nutrient requirement is dependent mainly on the quantity of milk secreted. The production capacity is an individual physiologic characteristic, which is influenced by the environment. Among the influences that tend to diminish the secretion of milk, and may even suppress it completely, are such emotional factors as excitement, fear and anxiety. Another factor we may call demand. The breast must be completely emptied at each nursing period if the secretion of milk is to the maintained. If the infant does not require the entire content, then removing the residual portion manually helps to assure continued secretion.

Another essential to maintenance of milk secretion is an adequate diet. Deficiencies in the food intake eventually may lead to a diminution in the quantity secreted and may even alter the composition.

The Recommended Allowances proposed by the Food and Nutrition Board were made on the basis of an average secretion of 850 ml of milk daily. The daily amounts recommended exceed those of any other period for women. Actually the quantity of milk secreted is markedly variable among individuals. On the average, the mother who is able to nurse her infant secretes around $\frac{1}{2}$ liter of milk in the first week or two, increasing to as much as 1 liter by the fifth month of lactation.

Energy

The added energy allowance for lactation recommended by the National Research Council is 1000 Cal. above that for a nonlactating woman of similar size and activity. The average energy value of human milk is 70 Cal. per 100 ml. If the secretion is 850 ml daily, 600 Cal. is accounted for in the milk itself, leaving 400 of the 1000 Cal. allowance for other uses.

There is question as to whether the actual process of milk formation needs sufficient energy to be measurable. An assessment of human needs during lactation indicates that most likely the physiological processes of with formation involve only a limited energy expenditure.

Insufficient energy in the diet may lead eventually to a diminished secretion of milk. Overfeeding, on the other hand, does not stimulate additional milk production and seems even in some cases to diminish the quantity.

The increase in the Recommended Allowances for lactation is not equally great for energy and the nutrients. As summarized in Fig. 16.3 the addition to the recommended caloric intake over that for women of 25 years is 48% whereas for calcium, protein, and vitamin A the increase is much greater than that. It means that the foods added to supply the additional Calories must of necessity provide generously those nutrients needed in increased amounts; milk, and eggs are examples of good supplementary foods.

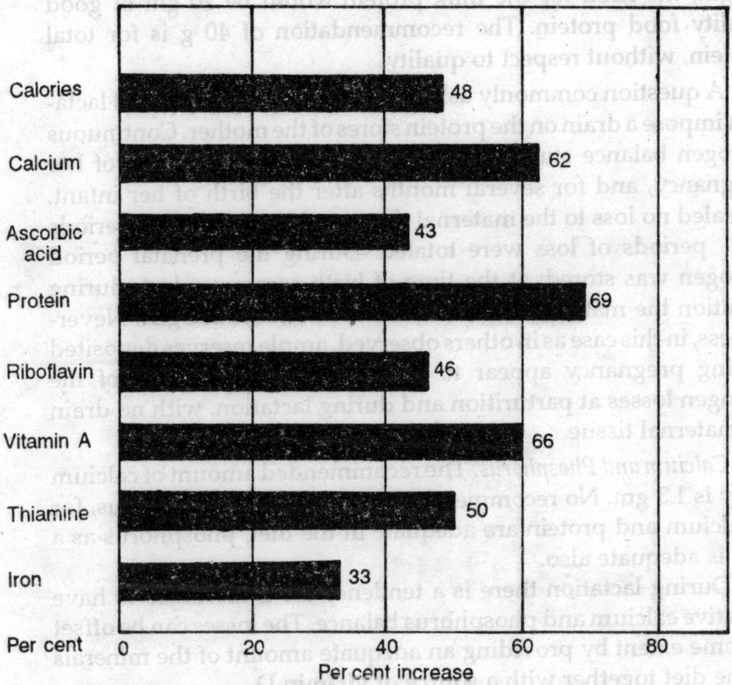

Fig. 16.3. Percentage increase in Recommended Allowances foe women during lactation, over allowances for women 25 years of age.

Protein

The Recommended Allowance for protein during lactation is a 20-gm daily increase over the recommendation for pregnancy and 40 gm greater daily than for the nonpregnant woman.

Inadequate protein in the diet generally causes diminution in the quantity of milk secreted. There is evidence that supplying sufficient protein during both pregnancy and lactation favours milk production.

At an international conference on protein requirements in 1957, it was proposed that about 2.0 gm of food protein of high nutritive value my be required to produce 1.0 gm of milk protein.

These values apply to women who have been consuming an adequate diet and not to those who are undernourished. If the amount of milk secreted is 850 ml, with a protein content of approximately 10 gm, the need for the milk protein would be 20 gm of good quality food protein. The recommendation of 40 g is for total protein, without respect to quality.

A question commonly asked is whether pregnancy and lactation impose a drain on the protein stores of the mother. Continuous nitrogen balance studies with one woman through most of her pregnancy, and for several months after the birth of her infant, revealed no loss to the maternal tissues when the storage periods and periods of loss were totaled. During the prenatal period nitrogen was stored; at the time of birth some was lost; during lactation the maternal tissues continued to lose nitrogen. Nevertheless, in this case as in others observed, ample reserves deposited during pregnancy appear to be sufficient to take care of the nitrogen losses at parturition and during lactation, with no drain on maternal tissue.

Calcium and Phosphorus: The recommended amount of calcium daily is 1.3 gm. No recommendation is made for phosphorus, for if calcium and protein are adequate in the diet, phosphorus as a rule is adequate also.

During lactation there is a tendency for individuals to have negative calcium and phosphorus balance. The losses can be offset to some extent by providing an adequate amount of the minerals in the diet together with a source of vitamin D.

Iron

Some iron is secreted in the milk, increasing the need to some extent for that element in the diet. The Food and Nutrition Board recommend that the allowance of 20 mg daily during pregnancy be continued through lactation.

The Vitamins

Less research has been done on the vitamin needs during lactation than for some of the other nutrients. The allowances proposed by the National Research Council, based on what research has been done and their own judgment, provides for sizable increases over the usual level for some of the vitamins. The actual amount needed by the mother is influenced by the quantity of milk produced.

The Recommended Allowances for the vitamins are: for vitamin A, 8000 IU daily, an increase of 60% over the allowance recommended for women 25 to 45 years of age; for thiamine, 1.2 mg, an increase of 50%; for riboflavin 1.9 mg, an increase of 46%; and for ascorbic acid 100 mg, an increase of 43%. For vitamin D the food and Nutrition Board recommend 400 IU, the same as far pregnancy. In support of their recommendation for vitamin D the state: "The optional amount of vitamin D for pregnancy and lactation is not known. On the basis of available evidence, 400 units is probably adequate."

16. 3. Nutrition of Older Persons

It is desirable that older persons enjoy freedom from handicaps that may have resulted from poor nutrition in their earlier years, or ill effects that may be caused by poor eating habits during their later life. As King explicitly states, "It is not enough to survive into the years from 60 to 80, they should be years of health and enjoyment, and mental vigor."

Concern for the nutrition of older people has continuously grown through the years, and justifiably so. The percentage of our population falling into the older age classification has progressively increased. Several factor have contributed to this change in the composition of the population. Among them are the increase in the number of births, which in turn results in more persons to grow old. Another influence, the decrease in death rate, has of course increased the number of older persons in the population.

Life expectancy at birth is predicted to increased by 45 to 50 per cent in 1975 over that observed in 1900. In Fig. 16.4 the life expectancy of women and men in 1900, 1950 and 1975 at birth, at age 45, and at age 65 are presented. The life expectancy for women is increasing more rapidly than for men.

Certain physiological changes that commonly accompany aging tend to decrease the functional capacity of the body. Changes that would be expected to have a direct effect on the utilization of food include a diminution in the size of the salivary glands, and a decrease in volume and acidity of gastric juice. Although there appears to little information on changes in the small intestine with advancing age, there is some evidence of a decreased rate of absorption. Furthermore, the colon appears to be unchanged. The

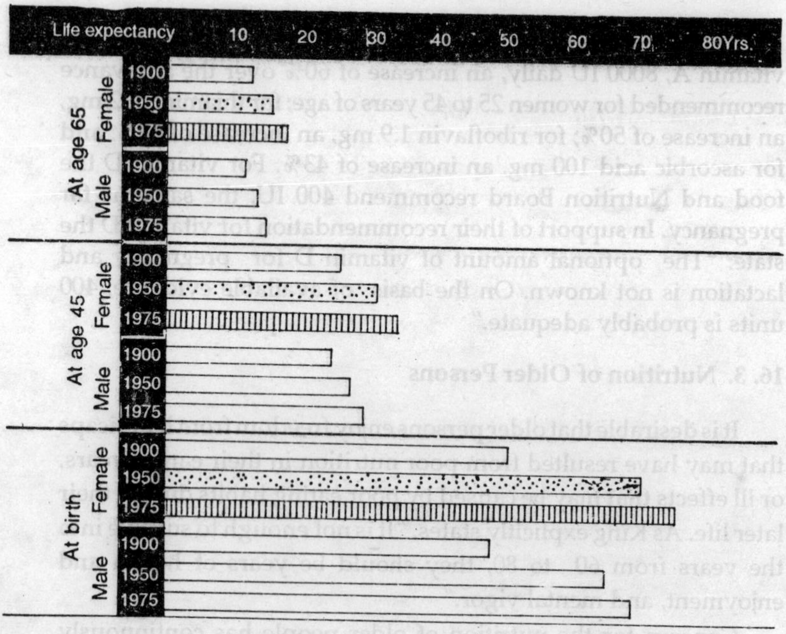

Fig 16.4. Increase in life expectancy for women and men.

gross weight of the liver decreases between the fourth and seventh decades. A common difficulty that hinders normal eating in older persons is the loss of teeth and failure to replace them with dentures.

There is evidence of less adequate carbohydrate metabolism in the older years. After consumption of a sugar solution (glucose tolerance test) or following a meal that was chiefly carbohydrate, older persons (men and women over 50 years) were found to have blood glucose values that were higher than that expected for younger adults. Stieglitz, who has been particularly concerned with the processes of aging in Individuals, explains that the "glucose tolerance test creates physiological stress" and with aging "tolerance for stresses of all sorts is diminished."

Nutrient Needs and Food Habits

Energy: In adults total energy needs decrease with aging. The Food and Nutrition Board proposes a 5% reduction in energy allowance per decade between ages 35 and 55 years; an 8%

reduction per decade from ages 55 to 75 years; and a further decrement of 10% is recommended for age 75 years and beyond. The daily Recommended Allowance for men 35 to 55 years of age is 2600 Cal.; for ages 55 to 75 years, 2200 Cal. For women 35 to 55 years of age the Daily Recommended Allowance is 1900 Cal.; for ages 55 to 75 years, 1600 Cal. The estimates are for persons normally active.

Factors that contribute to the decreasing energy need with aging are a lowered basal rate and the lessened physical activity that generally accompanies growing older. Causes for the progressive lowering of the basal rate, are not definitely known but are believed to be related to a combination of changes including (1) an alteration in body composition and (2) changes in the functioning of certain of the endocrine glands. With aging, the body tissues change in composition to relatively more fat and less muscular tissue. Estimates of the per cent of the body weight accounted for by fat in men ranging from 25 to 55 years of age are shown in Fig.16.5.

In actual practice, as people grow older they tend to eat less and thus compensate to some extent for the reduced energy needs. A problem that was common to persons whose diets were very low in energy value was the lowering of the nutrient content of

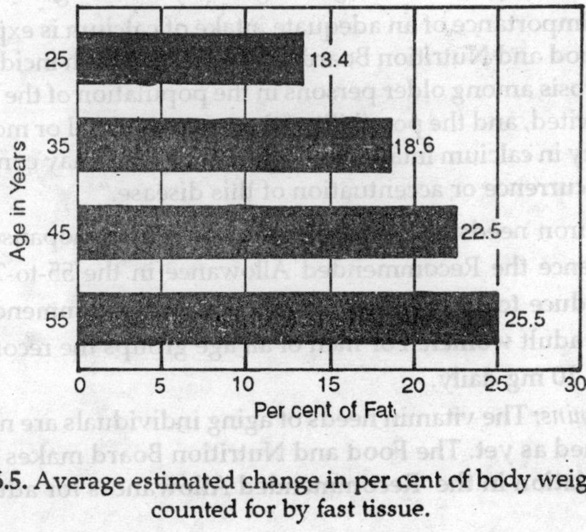

Fig. 16.5. Average estimated change in per cent of body weight accounted for by fast tissue.

the diet. However, the problem of too many Calories in the daily diet does exist because many of the older persons weighed more than accepted levels considered best for their health.

Protein: The protein needs of older person appears not to differ much from those of younger healthy adults. The Recommended Allowance is one gm per kg of body weight from young adulthood to old age, 18 to 75 years.

To supply the Recommended Allowance for protein, food relatively higher in protein content is required as persons grow older. This is necessary because the energy need decreases. At ages 55 to 75 years, the Recommended Allowance for protein provides 13 to 14 per cent of the total Calories whereas at ages 18 to 35 years only 10 to 11 per cent of the Calories are provided by protein.

Minerals: The mineral needs of older persons have not been studied to any great extent. As with energy and protein, the investigations of mineral need have been chiefly with women thus far. The Recommended Allowance for calcium for the 55-to-75 year age group is 0.8 gm daily, which is the same amount as recommended for younger adults. Calcium and phosphorus intakes, sufficient in amount that equilibrium between intake and outgo could be expected, were computed by Ohlson, using results from studies that she and others had done (*See* Table 16.1). The need for calcium as predicted by Ohlson is less after 70 years than in the preceding decades, beginning at 30 years of age.

The importance of an adequate intake of calcium is expressed by the Food and Nutrition Board. The relatively high incidence of osteoporosis among older persons in the population of the United States is cited, and the possibility "that even minimal or moderate deficiency in calcium intake over a period of years may contribute to the occurrence or accentuation of this disease."

The iron needs of women lessen after the menopause. As a consequence the Recommended Allowance in the 55-to-75 year age is reduce to 10 mg daily from the 15 mg recommended for younger adult women. For men of all age groups the recommendation is 10 mg daily.

Vitamins: The vitamin needs of aging individuals are not well established as yet. The Food and Nutrition Board makes no age differentiation in the Recommended Allowances for adults for

Table 16.1. Intakes of Calcium and Phosphorus Predicted for Equilibrium for Successive Decades in Women, 30 to 80 Years

Age Range, Years	No.	*Intake Predicted for Equilibrium* Calcium, gm/day	Phosphorus, gm/day
30-39	25	0.88	1.25
40-49	34	0.87	1.32
50-59	40	0.83	1.42
60-69	25	0.92	1.51
70-79	11	0.73	1.13

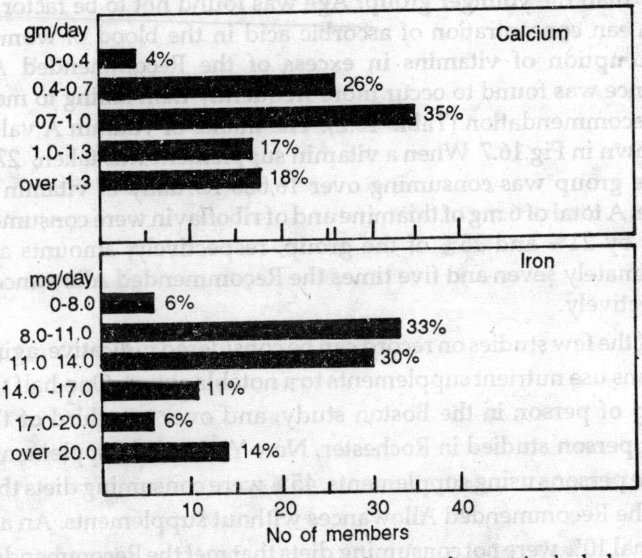

Fig. 16.6. Calcium and iron intake, supplement included.

vitamin A and ascorbic acid but does recommended a decrease in thiamine, riboflavin, and niacin equivalent with increasing age and the concomitant lower energy need. The Recommended Allowances for vitamin A ascorbic acid, thiamine, and riboflavin appear as a part of Table 16.2. For niacin equivalent the recommendation for men is 15 mg daily and for women 13 mg. There is evidence, however, that older women need more thiamine than younger women.

Table 16.2. Vitamin Intake of 104 Aging Persons

	Recommended Allowance		*Per Cent of Persons Consuming Vitamins at Various Levels*					
	Men	*Women*	*Amount*	*%*	*Amount*	*%*	*Amount*	*%*
Vitamin A value IU	5000	5000	4000-6999	21	>4000	7	<7000	70
Thiamine mg	0.9	0.8	1-2	32	>1	21	<2	49
Riboflavin mg	1.3	1.2	1-2	33	>1	3	<2	64
Ascorbic acid mg	70	70	50-100	30	>50	16	<100	17

At all levels of intake the excretion of thiamine was less for the older than the younger group. Age was found not to be factor in the mean concentration of ascorbic acid in the blood of women consumption of vitamins in excess of the Recommended Allowance was found to occur more frequently than failing to meet the recommendation (Table 16.2). The intake of vitamin A value is shown in Fig.16.7 When a vitamin supplement was taken, 27% of the group was consuming over 16,000 IU daily of vitamin A value. A total of 6 mg of thiamine and of riboflavin were consumed daily by 21% and 25% of the group, respectively, amounts approximately seven and five times the Recommended Allowances, respectively.

If the few studies on record can be considered indicative, aging persons use nutrient supplements to a notable extent. One-half the group of person in the Boston study, and over one-third of the older person studied in Rochester, New York used supplements. Of the persons using supplements, 45% were consuming diets that met the Recommended Allowances without supplements. An additional 10% were not consuming diets that met the Recommended Allowances in all nutrients, but even so the supplement did not provide the nutrients needed. Only of the 9.5% persons using supplements had preparations that provided all the nutrients needed to bolster the nutrient content of the diet.

16.4. Diet and Longevity

Experimental work with animals has demonstrated that kind and amount of food and manner of feeding have an influence on

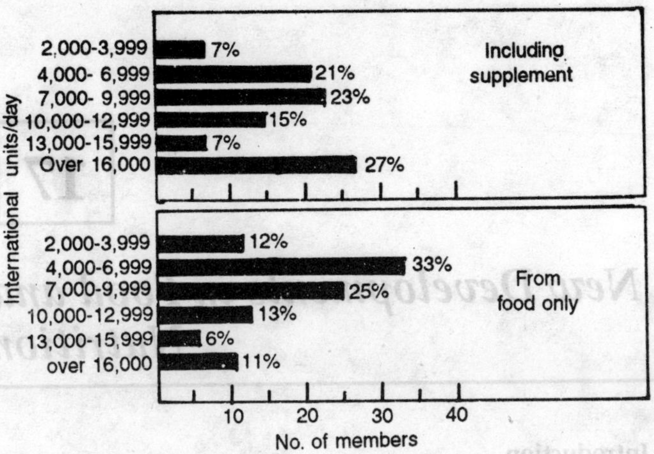

Fig. 16.7. Intake of vitamin A value.

length of life. Sherman, found that when diets adequate for growth and reproduction in the white rat were improved, the animals responded with increased growth, a prolonged reproductive period, and a longer life. The nutrients added were calcium, riboflavin and vitamin A.

Another approach to lengthening the life span through diet is that of retarding the rate of growth in young animals by limiting the caloric intake. McCay, fed diets planned to provide an abundance of food essentials but limited in energy value. Animals on this dietary regime grew slowly, matured atc and outlived the animals who ate an adequate diet ad libitum.

Alteration in the fat content of the diet tends to influence the life span of experimental animals. Rats fed a ration containing 22.7% fat had a shorter life span than those fed diets that were 3.4% fat. The two groups of animals grew at essentially the same rate.

These experimental studies on the relationship of diet to length of life are fundamental to our understanding of the far-reaching influence of diet on life processes. At present we do no see a direct application to human beings but, on the other hand, we do not summarily dismiss them as having no significance for man. Studies with the human take longer, particularly those concerned with longevity!

17

New Developments in Food and Nutrition

17.1. Introduction

In the discussion so far we have been considering the nutrients present in our food items, their needs, their functions their sources and the adverse effects of their deficiency etc. During last 30 years many new areas of research have emerged in foods and nutrition. The use of additives in foods has became a subject of national and international interest. Many a methods of food preservation have been developed strontuim-90 in the diet is one of the entirely new area for scientific investigation. The space probes by man has created a new research challenge for the food technologist, the physiologist, the biochemist and the nutritionist. In this chapter an attempt will be made to throw some light an hence topics.

17.2. Newer Methods of Food Presentation

Upto about the middle of nineteenth century the commonly used methods for preservation of food were *drylng, pickling, salting* etc. The process of preserving food by *cannying* was developed by *Francies* is in early 1800's. The process of freezing, which is now used to preserve both the raw and the processed food is a discovery of the twentieth century. Newer methods of food preservation include such methods as *dehydration, freeze drying* and *irradiation.*

Dehydrated Foods

The objective of dehydration is to remove most of the water from a food without changing its colour, flavour or texture.

Removal of moisture as a means of food preservation is one of the oldest of methods. Sun-drying of such foods as corns, apples and peaches was practiced in homes many a year ago and still is to same extent. Dehydration will doubtless continue to have limited usefulness as a means of holding foods for future use because of lack of public acceptance of same dehydrated foods.

The dehydrated foods of today, however, are quite superior to those of the past because of never methods of technology and moderns equipment. Different types of foods are presented by dehydration. Eggs, potatoes and their products, fruits, citrus fruit juices, soups and others.

The major advantages that the dehydrated foods have over fresh, canned or frozen counterparts are as follows:-

(i) They are economical

(ii) They are easy to prepare

(iii) They require no special equipment for storage

(iv) They are easy to transport.

Freeze-Dried Foods

The preservation method of freeze-drying involves the removal of water from a food by *sublimation* after it has been frozen. Sublimation is a physical process whereby a solid substance is vaporized or a vapor is condensed without first changing to a liquid. In freeze-drying, the frozen water or ice crystals in the food tissues vaporize and condense, leaving the tissues as water vapor without forming water.

Freeze-dried food products have several desirable qualities not found in food products dried from the liquid state (dehydration). They retain their natural shape, are least altered chemically, and are readily reconstituted with water.

Many types of foods have been subjected to the freeze-dried process on an experimental basis. However, until recently only limited numbers of these products have been sold for civilian use.

A comparison has been made between the taste of freeze-dried foods and the foods process by canning or freezing and it has been found that out of beef, pork, chicken, sea-foods, soup and some other mixtures of food those which were given a superior grading were beef, noodle soup, chicken noodle soup, and shirut, creole. Generally the score for frozen foods were higher when served as mixtures than when served plain.

Like dehydrated foods frozen foods also do not require any special equipment for storage, are easy to prepare and are economical to transport. But unlike dehydrated foods, they are expensive of not readily available.

Irradiated Foods

We all are familiar with x-rays as they can penetrate the body and are widely used in medical diagnostics. It radiation is similar to x-radiation and has similar power of radiation.

Just as the rays penetrate the body so they can penetrate food stuffs, and the principle behind radiation of food is to use the power of the rays to penetrate the food, while adjusting the dose of the rays so that germs are destroyed but the food staff itself not damaged in any way x-rays have very great power of penetration and can be used on sterilize food after it has been canned or packeted. It produces scarcely any heat and can be used on frozen food, such as poultry or frozen meat, without raising the temperature more than a degree or two. In fact radiation is possibly more effective at very low temperature and the dose can be reduced accordingly. It may be used to sterilize the foods completely though exact use of radiation is not known the possible use of radiations are to destroy spoilage germs and so to prolong the life of food and to destroy disease germs and so to make it safe to eat.

Radiation of foodstuffs probably represent a break through in food preservation, but for long time yet we must depend on traditional methods.

The irradiation process is sometimes referred to as "cold sterilization" because the microorganisms in the food are destroyed or inactivated by the nuclear ionization rather than by heat. In heat sterilization a food must be processed at about 240° F for an hour or more to produce a sterile product, whereas in irradiation the heat produced amount to only a small rise in temperature (not more than 10° C) for a very short period of time.

Doses of radiation used on foods are expressed by a unit called the *rad*, which represents 100 ergs of energy per gm of irradiated material.

In theory, radiation sterilization should provide a fresh or cooked sterile product with a better taste and texture than foods processed by heat sterilization. In practice, however, this does not always occur because large doses of radiation may produce marked off-flavours and changes in colour and texture in some foods. For example, foods may develop an off-flavor resembling a scorched taste, cooked meats may turn pink in color, and lettuce wilts.

Some of the undesirable effects of radiation on food can be controlled as follows:

(i) Offensive flavours and odours produced in meats and foods high in fats can be controlled by irradiation under vacuum or in an atmosphere of nitrogen.

(ii) During irradiation of milk the off flavours and metallic flowers can be eliminated by simultaneous irradiation and vacuum distillation.

Some of the loses that occur due to irradiation of food are as follows:

(i) The fat soluble vitamins (vitamins A, E and K) get destroyed where as absorbic acid, thiamine and phyridoxine are reduced to about the same level as in processing by heat sterilization.

No evidence could be found of toxicity from eating irradiated foods.

It appears that small or medium doses of ionizing radiation may have a more immediate application to food preservation than the large dose of "cold sterilization" technique. Small doses of radiation (less than 100 thousand rads) have been used successfully to deinfest flour and spices, to prevent sprouting in stored potatoes, and to delay the ripening of fruit (Table 17.1). The same treatment may have a significant use to destroy the organism in pork that causes trichinosis. Medium doses of radiation (about 100 thousand to 1 million rads) now referred to as "pasteurization" or "radiopasteurization" have been shown to extend the shelf life of some foods stored under refrigeration. Meats have had their shelf life increased fivefold when treated with 100 to 500 thousand rads. Fruits treated with 100 to 150 thousands rads, packed under vacuum, and stored at refrigerator temperature were quite acceptable for a period of four or five months.

Table 17.1 The Use and Effect of Varying Levels of Ionizing Radiation on Food and Related Products

Level of Ionizing Radiation	*Use*	*Effect of Finished Product*
Small Exposure (less than 100 thousand rads)	Prevents sprouting of potatoes, destroys insects in flour and spices, and delays ripening of fruit.	Products not sterile but little or no effect on flavor
Medium Exposure or "Pasteurization" (about 100 thousand to 1 million rads)	Extends the shelf life of meats, fish, fruits, and vegetables under refrigeration.	Products not completely sterile but little or no effect on flavor or color of foods.
Large Exposure or "Sterilization" (a few million rads)	Sterilizes foods so they can be stored as canned foods when properly packaged.	Products completely sterile but often causes marked off-flavors and changes in colour and texture.

17.3. Additives to Foods

Marry foods items marketed these days have had chemicals added. These chemicals, added to food are known as *food additives.* A food additive can be defined as, "a substance or a mixture of substances, other than basic food stuff, which is present in food as a result of any aspect of production, processing, storage or packaging."

Although some of the substances are introduced intentionally for the purpose of improving the nutritive value or quality of the product, others are present as a residue after some stage of production or manufacture. The latter type of substance is essential in modern agricultural production and food technology.

Additives to Improve Nutritive Value

Some of the nutrients are added to food so as to improve their nutritive value. The first such additive was Iodine to salt that was done for the first time in 1924. The next important additive of this type was the increasing of vitamin D content of milk by adding irradiated ergosterol. Next one in the series may be considered as the enrichment of white flour and bread, in 1941, with the addition of specified amounts of thiamine, riboflavin, niacin and iron, and the addition of specified amount of vitamin D and calcium were optional. In 1947 these substances were used to enrich cores meal and corn grits. Now a days rice is also enriched. Margarine may be fortified with vitamin A and its concentration must be equivalent to 15.000 IU of the vitamin her bound which is approximately the same as the vitamin A potency of butter.

It should be kept in mind that bolstering the nutritive value of staple foods, beneficial as it may be, is not a substitute for education in the proper choice and preparation of foods. It is wise to continuously exert effort toward improving methods of production, processing, and storage, attempting to preserve more fully the nutrients present in the native products.

Increasing in use, particularly in beverages, are non-nutritive sweeteners as sugar substitutes (1). Saccharin and the calcium and sodium cyclamates (cyclohexyl sulfamates) are commonly used. Such sweeteners were permitted in foods in the first place for persons who needed to restrict their intake of carbohydrate. Now widespread use has been made of the products by persons who wish to reduce caloric intake.

Additives to Improve the Quality of Products

As the processing of foods became more complicated there arises a greater need for the additives. For any lighly processed food to be acceptable in keeping quality, flavor and standard characteristics, the addition of certain Chemical is essential.

We add *ascorbic acid* to some fruit is order to prevent their browning during the process of freezing.

We add *sulfur dioxide* to dried apricots and apples to prevent their discolouration.

Emlusifiers are added to bakery products is order to improve volume, uniformity and fineness of grain.

Emulsifiers are also added to confectionery for homogeneity and keeping quality. They are also added to dairy products for smoothness.

Commonly used emulsifiers are lecitheis, the mono-and di-glycerides, prophylene glycol, chemists generally refers to emulsifiers as 'surfactants' because of the fact that they surface acting agents.

Some *preservatives* are also added to extend and keep the quality of the product.

Antioxidants such as butylated hydroxyanisode (BHA), butylated hydroxy toluene (BHT), nordihydroguariaretic acid (N D G A) and propyl gallate, are added to fats so as to delay the onset of rancidity.

Preservatives used in bread are known as *rope inhibitors* or *anticycolic agents*. Preservatives permitted for bread include sodium propionate, calcium propionate, sodium, diacetate, acetic acid, lactic acid and monocalcium phosphate.

For cheese the antimycotic agents used are sorbic acid and potassium sorbates Those preservatives that prevent those physical or chemical changes which affect colour, flavor, texture, or appearance are known as *sequestrants*. Those used in dairy products include sodium, calcium, and potassium salts of citric, tartaric, metaphosphoric, and pyrophosphoric acids. Other common preservatives are benzoic acid, sodium benzoate, sulfur dioxide, sugar, salt, and vinegar.

Stabilizers and thickeners are used so as to improve smoothness of texture of confectionery, ice cream, and other frozen desserts; uniformity of colour, flavor, and viscosity of chocolate milk; "body" of artificially sweetened beverages. Stabilizing and thickening agents include pectins vegetable gums (carob bean, carragheen, guar), gelatin, and agar agar.

Acids, alkalies, buffers, and neutralizing agents are added to influence the degree of acidity or alkalinity, which is important in many classes of processed foods. For example, the acid ingredient acts on the leavening agent in baked goods, and releases the gas which causes rising. The taste of many soft drinks is due to an organic acid. Acidity of churning cream must be controlled for flavor and keeping quality of the butter. Acids contribute flavor to confectionery and help to prevent a "grainy" texture. Buffers and neutralizing agents are chemicals that are added to control acidity or alkalinity, just as acids and alkalies may be added directly. Some common chemicals in this class are ammonium bicarbonate, calcium carbonate, potassium acid tartarate, sodium aluminum phosphate and tartaric acid.

Flavoring agents are added to improve the taste in such products like soft drinks, bakery goods, confectionery, and ice cream. Synthetic flavors are provided by such chemicals as amyl acetate, Benzaldehyde, carvone, ethyl butyrate, and methyl salicylate.

Coloring matter is added to improve the appearance. These additives are introduced with no concern for nutritive value but with concern for the quality of the product, which of course influences the consumers' choice.

Incidental Additives

Incidental additives are those chemical substances that remain in foods from some stage of production of manufacture of the product. The most important additives in this classification are the "pesticides." Included in this general grouping are insecticides, fungicides, and rodenticides, each of which helps in the control of pests harmful to crops and food. Through the use of these chemicals, the production of food is facilitated; there is less loss of crops and food during storage; also the product produced is of higher quality.

In use of the additives there are various dangers and the law places responsibility on the manufacturers to demonstrate that the residues are harmless under conditions of use. Thus in case of commercially canned or frozen foods, the processor is responsible for using products that comply with the established tolerances.

"As an administrative principle, tolerances are set by FDA at 1/100 of the lowest level which causes effects in the most sensitive test animals whenever data on human toxicity are not available" (15, p. 17). In the case of some pesticides no amount of residue is permitted because of their high toxicity; for others no tolerances are established because the residues are harmless.

The law requires that chemicals for use in processing food must be proved by the industry to be safe for that purpose *before* they can be sold. The manufacturer or promoter of a new food additive must test it for safety on animals and submit the results to the Food and Drug Administration. If the Food and Drug

Administration is satisfied as to the safety of the additive, it will issue a regulation specifying the amount which may be used, the foods in which it may be used. If the safety of the additive is not established, its use will be prohibited.

Keeping in view the international problem of food additives, World Health Organization Committee on Food additives was established in 1955. It has been dealing mainly with the evaluation of "the evidence on the toxicological aspects of a number of antimicrobials and antioxidants used as food additives". Such substances "are widely used in many countries, because they can play an important part in reducing food wastage by improving storage efficiency and distribution...." In some countries there are departments responsible for the control of the use of these drugs. "In many others, however, there is no adequate machinery by which those responsible for public health can usefully handle these problems."

Its recommendations about baby foods given in 1961 says, "baby foods should be prepared without food additives if possible" If not possible, it was urged that, "great caution should be exercised both in the choice of the additive and in the level of use". This special consideration for infants can be explained an the basis that, "the detoxicating mechanism that are effective in more mature individuals may be in effective in the baby."

17.4. Strontium-90 in the Diet

One of the hazardous by-products of fission piles and atomic blasts is the radioactive form of strontium-90. This contamination product may be a potential cause of sarcomas in the animal organism. Because of the long half-life of this "bone-seeking" radionuclide (about 28 years) there is a worldwide interest in the preset rates of strontium-90 accumulation in plants, and man due to the contamination of the earth's atmosphere from bomb tests within recent years.

Since strontium is a member of the alkaline earth metals group and so it has a similarity in behaviour to calcium. Both minerals move in the "food chain" from soil to plant to animal to man. Both get deposited in bones and teeth. However in the animal organism, there is a preferential absorption of calcium then that of strontium from the body. Their biological preference is used to protect the body against the accumulation of excess of strontium.

Man ingests amounts of strontium in the food he eats because it is one of the trace elements normally found in biological material. Harrison and his group have reported that from a normal diet their subjects ingested about 1.99 mg of strontium per day and excreted nearly the same amount (about 1.97 mg per day). The body load of strontium in man has been demonstrated to be about four to six times higher after an intravenous dose than after an oral dose.

Radiostrontium in the Diet

Strontium-90 is measured in units known as *micromicrocuries* (μμc) or *picocuries* (pc). The Food Protection Committee of the National Research Count has suggested that the values for dietary strontium-90 be expressed in two ways: the amount of strontium-90 per unit of Calcium and the amount of stronium-90 per unit product. For example, the 1959 wheat crop grown in the United States averaged about 113 μμc (or pc) or strontium-90 per gm of calcium and 46 μμc (or pc) of strontium-90 per kg of wheat.

For almost a decade, the Health and Safety Laboratory of the Atomic Energy Commission, the United States Public Health Service, and other research units in that country have conducted regular analyses for strontium-90 and other radionuclides in the American food and water supply. Data from similar analyses are available from other parts of the world.

Indices of the strontium-90 content of the food supply at any one time are determined in several ways. One procedure is to use the radioactivity in milk as a guide to strontium-90 in the diet, another procedure is to present data in terms of amounts of food typical for various age groups, and a newer approach is to present data in terms of the food need for the group with the largest nutritive requirement in the population (the male teenager).

The average values of strontium-90 ranged from 13 to 4.3 μμc per gram of calcium. Although methods have been suggested and developed for the remedial modification of foods to remove radiostrontium but the committee on food has stated, "the present extent of environmental contamination does not warrant extra-ordinary measures for the decontamination of foods."

16.5. Food and Nutriture for Man in Space

History undoubtedly will record the research and development directed to the accomplishment of manned space flight as one of the greatest scientific and engineering feats of all times.

The manned balloon flights conducted prior to the suborbital and orbital flights of Project Mercury gave significant information on man's performance at high altitudes. It was found that man could exist for more than a day in sealed cabin at high altitudes, approximately 100,000 feet (19 miles) in the atmosphere. These pioneer test pilots breathed are artificial atmosphere and ate a ration composed of specially prepared foods.

Some Studies Directed to Nutriture for Space Travel

In the following paragraphs a brief outline of some of the studies about the nutriture for man's exploration of space are taken up. Tubed foods, freeze-dried foods, unconventional-type foods, equipment for feeding the space traveler, and feeding concepts for Projects Mercury and Gemini are presented in very brief.

Tubed Foods: These types of food products were developed for personnel performing in high-flying aircraft and space vehicles where pressure suits and other conditions might interfere with normal feeding procedures. Tubed foods can be eaten without the removal of a pressure helmet, do not require refrigeration, are ready to eat, are not affected by high altitudes, and need little storage and disposal space.

The food, either in the liquid or semisolid form, is packed in a pliable aluminum tube to which is fitted a screw-on, five-inch plastic tube known as a pontube. When the tube is squeezed by hand, food passes into the mouth via the pontube. Welbourn and Lachance have measured the palatability of nineteen different tubed foods with human subjects. The twelve tubed foods found to warrant consideration for operational use were applesauce, peaches, vegetable juice, fruit dessert, semisolid beef, chocolate, semisolid chicken, pork dinner, semisolid ham, veal dinner, beef dinner, and beef noodle soup.

Freeze-dried Foods: The proposed use of freeze-dried foods in the fourteen-day flights of Project Gemini and Apollo has given impetus to an intensive research and development programme of this type of food preservation. Details on freeze-dried food products are presented in preceding article.

Unconventional Types of Foods: The need to supply adequate nutrition in future long-range space flights, where it no longer will be possible to carry sufficient supplies for life support, has led to the initiation of studies to find unconventional food products that can be used as sources of Calories, amino acids, minerals, and vitamins for the space traveler. Although bacteria and vegetable tissues grown in tissue cultures have been proposed as "potential space food" the two examples of unconventional food sources presented here are the high energy metabolites and algae.

High-energy metabolites are long-chained compounds which have a caloric value greater than that of the conventional energy nutrients: carbohydrate, 4 Cal. per gm; fat, 9 Cal. per gm; and protein, 4 Cal. per gm. Two high-energy metabolites now under study are 1. 3-butanediol and 2, 4-dimethyl heptanoic acid. It has been reported that in diets of rats, 1, 3-butanediol was utilized for energy at about 6 Cal. per gm to replace dietary carbohydrate and to increase the caloric density of high-fat rations.

The use of algae as a food supplement is not new. People in various parts of the world, specially in the Far East, have used small portions of algae in their diets for centuries. There are various kinds of algae: green, blue-green, red and brown. In general, a 100-gm portion of powdered green algae contains about 59 gm of protein, 19 gm of fat, 13 gm of carbohydrate, and 550 Cal. Analytical data in terms of protein, amino acids, certain vitamins, lipids, ash, and energy in various algae and mixture of algae have been reported.

There is interest in this unicellular plant for space travel because of its photosynthetic properties where-by algae may be useful both as a food and a respiratory gas exchanger. In the process of photosynthesis, carbon dioxide is used by the plant to synthesize nutrients, and oxygen is produced as a by-product in these reactions. Thus the carbon dioxide of the expired air may be exchanged for oxygen in this cycle. Also there is considerable interest in the possible production and use of algae in the over-populated countries of the world to bolster the nutritive value of their inadequate food supplies.

Although may studies have been conducted on the culture and growth of algae, the use of the plant in algae gas exchange systems, the composition of algae , and other related topics, data on the acceptability and tolerance of algae feeding in man are scare. In a study the algae, a mixture of *Chlorella* and *Scenedesmus,* was added to the basal diet in increasing amounts during the six-week period of the study. In an attempt to mask the strong, bitter taste of the algae, the plant product was incorporated into such foods as gingerbread, chocolate cookies, and chocolate cake. It was found that algae intakes up to a level of 100 gm per day, incorporated into the basal diet, were tolerated by all subjects. Early in the study, however, some of the subjects manifested gastrointestinal symptoms which increased at algae intakes above 100 gm per day. Some subjects experienced headaches, vomiting, and malaise at these higher levels of intake. Despite the reduced tolerance of algae at levels above 100 gm per day, no abnormalities were detected by either the physical or the clinical measurements in this study.

It has been suggested that some of the poor acceptability and lack of tolerance associated with algae as a food may be related to bacterial contamination. They have found that in a "self-nourishing" (autotrophic) algae culture as much as one-third of the culture population may be bacteria.

Work is now under way to investigate the potential of decolourized algae as a food source. The strong taste and odor of green algae can be removed to yield a product quite bland in taste and odor. However, the nutrient value of decolourized algae has not been reported so far.

In addition to the work with algae, there is an interest in the possible use of higher plants as food sources for the permanent space stations of the future. Some of the plants being studied are cabbage, cauliflower, Chinese cabbage, dandelion, endive, kale, lettuce, sweet, potato and tampala.

Equipment for Feeding the Space Traveler: Many types of equipment have been designed, fabricated, and tested for the purpose of feeding man during high-altitude flight and space travel. A plastic water-container, a feeding system using aluminium cans, a solar-powered oven, and feeding ports for tubed foods are just a few examples of types of feeding equipment that have been developed. Of special interest is the development and evolution of the design of the feeder and dispenser used for space feeding.

The Life Support System and Feeding Concept of Project Mercury

One of the important research areas in the Manned Space Programme has been and still is the undertakings directed to provide the astronaut with an adequate life support balance from the time he leaves until he returns to earth.This balance includes the life support needs for pressure, oxygen, water, as well as food, and the removal of the products of metabolism (carbon dioxide, water, heat, urine and feces).

An outline sketch of the general features of the life support system used in the space flights of Project Mercury is shown in Fig. 17.1 Because of the need to conserve weight and space in these initial space flights, a supply of oxygen and water was carried in these missions for the closed environmental system designed for Project Mercury. In this type of system the astronaut wore a pressure suit continually, ventilated with 5 pounds per square inch of oxygen in the pressurized cabin of the vehicle. The end products of metabolism were collected and treated in the following way: carbon dioxide was removed by absorption with lithium hydroxide; water was removed by a water separator, and that condensed in the heat exchanger removed mechanically; heat was removed by a water-evaporative heat exchanger; odors were absorbed by activated charcoal; urine was collected in a device worn

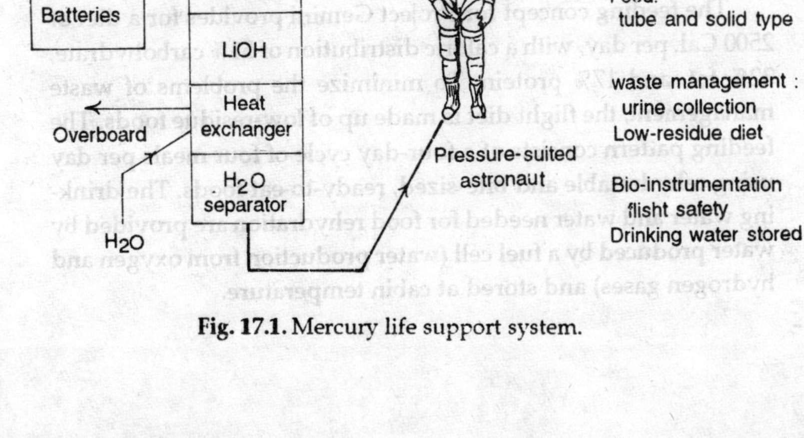

Fig. 17.1. Mercury life support system.

in the pressure suit; and fecal product was controlled by the ingestion of a low-residue preflight diet.

For the Project Mercury flights no food was carried on board the spaceships in the first two short-time suborbital flights. In the later orbital flights, however, the handling of food and food containers was an experimental phase of the flight plan and information was also collected on gastrointestinal function during periods of weightlessness. The food items used in the early orbital flights were pureed foods (meats, vegetables and fruits), malted milk tablets, and bite-size food cubes. Dehydrated foods were included in the food pattern of flight MA-9.

The Feeding Concept of Russian Spaceflights

Little information is available on the feeding concept used in the Russian spaceflights. However, facts concerning Russian space feeding as found in documents from the Library of Congress are as follows:

Gargarin and Titov, the first of the Russian cosmonauts, ingested pureed foods from tubes in their flights into space. The space diets of Nikolayev and Popovich contained ordinary-type foods (i.e., meat cutlets, fried veal, chicken fillet, and sandwiches) prepared in small pieces as well as tubed foods. Water, coffee, and fruit juices have been reported to have complemented the semi-solid and bite-sized foods of the space ration. Large doses of vitamins also were important in the Russian space diet. The space feeding pattern of the Russian cosmonauts appears to be a scheduled food intake every four or five hours.

The Feeding Concept of Project Gemini

The feeding concept for Project Gemini provides for a diet of 2500 Cal. per day, with a caloric distribution of 51% carbohydrate, 32% fat, and 17% protein. To minimize the problems of waste management, the flight diet is made up of low-residue foods. The feeding pattern consists of a four-day cycle of four meals per day using rehydratable and bite-sized, ready-to-eat foods. The drinking water and water needed for food rehydration are provided by water produced by a fuel cell (water production from oxygen and hydrogen gases) and stored at cabin temperature.

18

Improvement of Already-Normal Nutrition

18.1. Introduction

These days health is not merely the absence of disease but a positive quality of life which can be build to higher levels. We now make a clear distraction between merely adequate nutrition and the optimum nutrition. Now we talk of expected potentialities of nutritional improvement of life that has become a reality because of various advances in research methods.

18.2. Increasingly Comprehensive Methods of Research

In various research methods towards nutritional problems which have to be directed for life times and even successive generations, the following two kinds of experimental variables are chosen :

(*i*) *The individual chemical factor* or compound.

(*ii*) *The article of food* as produced by nature or agriculture.

By 1930 it had been shown that a dietary made up of everyday food materials may be permanently adequate to the needs of normal nutrition, including those of growth, reproduction, and lactation, generation after generation, and yet that nutritional well-being and length of life may be improved by a more scientific adjustment of the everyday foods in the dietary.

In his work Auden (1923) of Birmingham, England, found that not only poorly nourished or undernourished but also "supposedly adequately nourished children," responded to the feeding of extra milk with increased gains in body weight and hemoglobin and "an improvement in bodily and mental vigor."

Mann (1922-26) carried out experiments an English school boys with very precise and accurate measurements he showed that boys, who were already normally nourished at the start, made better gains in both height and weight when milk (and, in lesser degree, when watercress) was added to their accustomed diet. As the milk clearly gave better increments of gain than any of the other supplements tested, repeated comparisons of the normal diet with and without the extra milk were made. The results proved beyond doubt a better physical and mental growth in the boys getting the extra milk (though the diet without it was already supporting normal nutrition). Some other experimenters have also concluded that alertness and mental growth and performance, as well as growth in physique, were improved by addition of extra milk, from a starting point of already-normal nutrition.

From numerous studies carried out by various researchers it has now become clear that starting with already-normal nutrition, both mental and physical growth and development can be improved by superior selection and proportioning of the everyday foods in the diet.

Findings have also revealed that in case of adults, the larger the proportion of "protective" food in the diet, the smaller was the proportion of failures in the preservation of the characteristics of youth.

In the chemical laboratory of Columbia University, it was found as already noted, that a mixture of five sixths ground whole wheat and one sixth dried whole milk, with pure table salt and distilled water, which we may call *Diet* A, was *adequate* in that it supported (in experiments with rats) normal growth and health with successful reproduction and rearing of young, generation after generation.

Yet when the proportion of milk was increased, to constitute *Diet B*, the average results were *better*. And, as we now know, *Diet B* is capable of further improvement. Such experiments, dealing with problems of improvement of already- adequate diets, and of already-normal nutrition, have no (1951- 52) been carried on continuously for over twenty years and have repeatedly furnished objective evidence of the improvability of already-normal nutrition. Good judges readily agreed that better nutrition of babies contributes to the making of better babies; but acceptance of a corresponding nutritional improvement of the norm among adults (or improvement of the adult life expectation) came more slowly because it had been supposed that "longevity depends on heredity."

With the development of today's better criteria and techniques of life-time and successive-generation experiments with laboratory animals, we can now study the effects of food upon life history, both qualitatively and quantitatively, as in the work with Diets A and B mentioned above.

Change in Proportions of Natural Foods

From the results of the above experiments Diet A and Diet B it was objectively and conclusively proved that already-normal nutrition can still be nutritionally improved and that a shift in proportions of everyday foods may measurably improve the nutritive value of already adequate Diet A.

If we compare Diet A with Diet B are find that the only difference between than is in the relative proportions of wheat and milk but the change of this proportion made Deity B richer than Diet A in four individual (chemical) nutrients. There was small increasing protein content but larger increases in Calcium, vitamin A and riboflavin.

It has to be always kept in mind that there may be still undiscovered substances essential to nutrition.

Higher Intakes of Calcium and of Vitamin A

Further experimentation was done with diets differing in their calcium contents only to the same extent as in the above mentioned mixtures of natural food materials. This increase of calcium intake (from 0.2 to 0.34 - 0.4% of the air-dry food mixture) resulted in slightly more rapid growth, more efficient utilization of food value (whether computed in terms of calories or of proteins), slightly earlier maturity, better success in reproduction and lactations some increase in average length of adult life. The gain in longevity by males was significant while that by females was less. However, females who received more calcium had borne and reared more young.

Further studies also revealed that

(*i*) increase of calcium intake did increase the longevity of animated females, (*ii*) increase of calculating intake resulted in both increased success in reproduction and lactation and attainment of greater longevity by females.

With calcium intakes somewhat higher than of Diet B (see Table 18.1) the average lengths of adult life were increased 10.4% in males and 13.8% in the females as compared with Diet A. *With increased vitamin A intake,* males lived 10.1% and females 12.1% longer than on the Diet A described above on which rat families have repeatedly thrived for 70 to 75 generations.

Table 18.1. Influence of Food Upon Attainment of Definite Ages by Rats

Percentage of Lives Longer than	*Males*		*Females*	
	On Diet A	*On Diet B*	*On Diet A*	*On Diet B*
600 days	42.9	65.3	54.1	73.0
700 days	14.8	32.3	27.6	43.6
800 days	2.9	10.5	12.2	15.9
900 days	0.0	1.6	1.6	5.5
1000 days	0.0	0.0	0.5	1.2

It has already been pointed out in our discussion on vitamins that increased intake of vitamin A yield increasingly beneficial results of intake upto about four times the minimal adequate level. Further experiments have established that vitamin A is a significant factor along with calcium and riboflavin in nutritional improvement of an already adequate diet by simple shifting of the proportions of natural foods. The results have shown that extra intake of vitamin A specially influences the maintenance of high health and low death rates in the older adults. However, it remains to be seen what life histories would result from comprehensive tests of diets carrying optional enrichments both of calcium and vitamin A and from changes of diet at different points of the life history.

Ascorbic Acid (Vitamin C)

The increased intake of vitamin C bring increased benefits upto the levels 5-6 times as high as needed for simple prevention of scurvy.

Riboflavin: Increased intake of riboflavin has been found to confer increasingly beneficial results upto the intake levels twice as high as that of minimal edequacy of permanently normal nutrition. Any further increase seems to confer additional benefit upon the off springs. Thus the benefit to the internal environment of the mothers body is more delicately reflected in her off spring than in her own adult organism.

To provide a better and filler chemical explanation may be possible by the combined results of

(*i*) studies of molecular structures of the tissues enzymes and coenzymes and the exact nature of the chemical reactions which they catalyze, and

(*ii*) Determination of riboflavin and related factors in off spring of differently fed experimental animal families at early ages by improved methods.

While, the zone between the minimal-adequate and optimal levels of intake is not equally wide for all nutrients, and calcium, riboflavin, and vitamins A and C were not taken at rondom for the comprehensive investigations here mentioned but were especially studied because of the promise of earlier work with natural foods. It is clear that the recent studies of the kind reveal previously unexpected degrees of potentiality in the improvement of already normal health and efficiency through a more scientifically guided daily use of food.

Now it can be said that the newer knowledge of nutrition offers man a longer lease of healthier life than has before been enjoyed by any but only a fortunate few.

Nature and Nurture

Both quality and length of life are greatly influenced by heredity and nutrition. Evidence is available to show that liberal use of protective foods may serve to diminish the incidence of, or severity, or duration of other diseases as also the nutritional diseases.

Present day medical view emphasizes that the nutritional background and foundation afforded by the habitual use of a dietary which is thoroughly well-balanced, with reference to the newly discovered as well as longer-known factors, may greatly advance the probability of a satisfactory outcome of whatever medical measure is to be undertaken.

Table 18.2. Influence of Diet on Rate of Growth and Length of Life

Rats of Columbia University Department of Chemistry Colony, 1920—1950

	Rate of Growth	*Length of Life*	*Useful Life*	*Reference*
Increased proportion of milk in already adequate diet (Diet A)	Increased	Increased	Increased	Sherman and Campbell, 1924, 1928, 1930
Addition of butterfat to Diet A	Decreased	Increased	Increased	Sherman and Campbell, 1937
Addition of skim milk solids to Diet A	Increased	Increased	Increased	"
Addition of Calcium to Diet A	Increased	Increased	Increased	"
Doubling the vitamin A of Diet A without adding appreciable fat	Increased	Increased	Increased	Campbell, Udiljak, Yarmolinsky, and Sherman, 1945
Again doubling vitamin A	Unchanged	Increased	Increased	Sherman and Trupp, 1949
Increase of calcium from 0.2 to 0.64% in diet	Increased	Increased	Increased	Van Duyne, et al. 1941
Diversification of diet of natural foods	Increased	Unchanged	Slightly increased	Campbell and Sherman, 1938
Increase of protein from 16% to 20% of the food	Increased	Unchanged	Slightly increased	Sherman, Campbell, and Ragan, 1949
Increase of protein from 14% to 24% of the food	Increased	Doubtful [a]	Doubtful [a]	Sherman, Pearson, and Bal, 1950

Furthermore it has been established that in case of a given individual, family or community, the superior nutritional well-being induced by taking a higher proportion of food as protective food favours the efficiency of brain as also of the other organs.

The fate of growth does not necessarily influence the length of life can be seen from the findings on fats of Coulumbia University Department of chemistry (Table 18.2).

In this scientific world, which expects progress, the shortness of individual lives tends to set a limit to the actual use by man of the knowledge which he has accumulated and the institution which he has built and developed. Hence the longer term of fully efficient years which the newer chemistry of food and nutrition offer may be of exceedingly far-reaching significance to human progress. Late President Wood Ward once remarked that the third of a professional or scientific man's years pass by the time he finishes his formal schooling and probably another one-third is spent in proving himself of utility to the society and thus he is left with only one-third of his years for rendering his fullest service to the world. This pattern of life behaviour tallies will if we study the life histories of some famous scientists of our times.

Thus there are various advantages, to the individual and to the society, from the earlier attainment and longer retention of the full adult capacity and efficiency of the people who receive the benefits of the new knowledge of nutrition.

We should always keep in mind that when superior nutriton increases the length of life this is only one expression of the fact that life has been lived on a higher level of health and efficiency through out. For an individual, it means more years in prime life and not in old age. For the nation, it means larger percentage of population consists of such people who are mature and still of full economic, cultural and social value.

So far there is only beginning of adequate appreciation of the fact that the body's "steady states" are only relatively so, and that we have power to improve both the quality and the duration of life by cultivation such food habits as help to keep the concentration of each nutrient (in the internal environment or fluid matrix) at such level as is found by research to be most conducive to well-being.

Nutritional improvement of life advances the prospect for achievement of our ideals whatever these may be.

The present is, and the near future undoubtedly will be, a period of important opportunity in the advancement of human welfare through the increase, and the diffusion, and the practical application, of nutritional knowledge. Some important things which science previously thought to be beyond its power, it is now learning to accomplish through the newer chemistry of food and nutrition.